WIN THE FIGHT

STOMP OUT MELANOMA

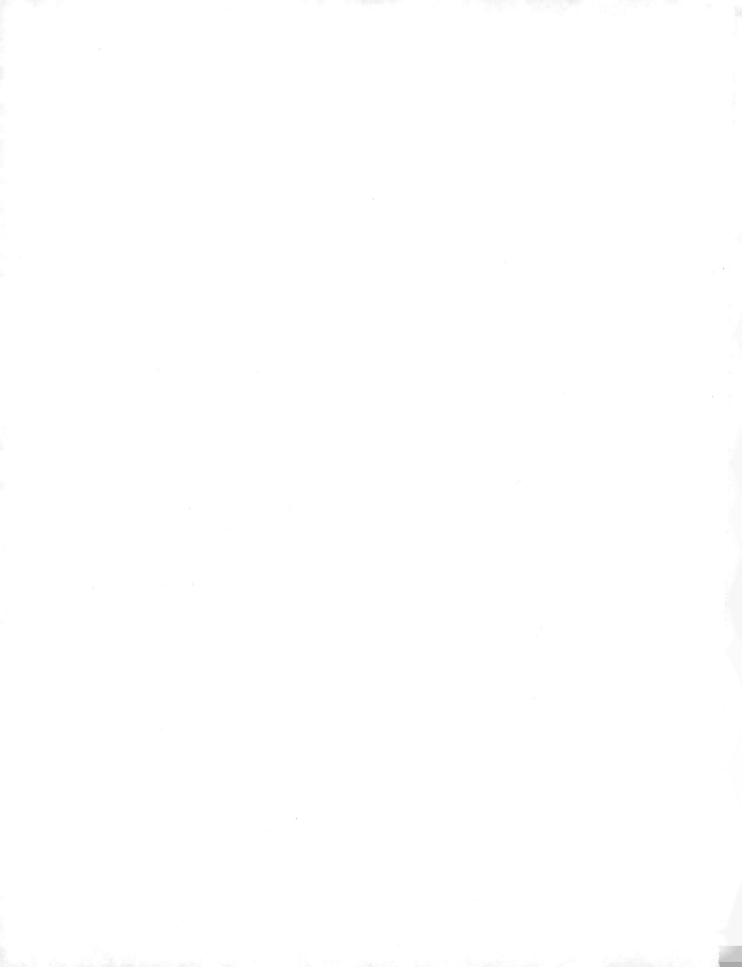

WIN THE FIGHT

STOMP OUT MELANOMA

How to **WIN THE FIGHT**
against melanoma and maximize your cancer
treatment with holistic nutrition, exercise,
and stress reduction

Deepak Narayan, MD
Melanoma Specialist

Lisa Lynn PT
Fitness & Nutrition Expert

Illustrations by Deepak Narayan & Joseph Cuticelli

A portion of the proceeds from the sale of this book will be used to fund melanoma research

WIN THE FIGHT: Stomp Out Melanoma
Deepak Narayan and Lisa Lynn

Printed in the United States of America

ISBN: 978-0-9908216-2-5

DEDICATION

This book is designed and dedicated to all cancer survivors, caretakers/caregivers and their loved ones who make the fight worthwhile. Just as importantly, the team of medical professionals who dedicate their lives to helping people fight back every day.

It is their journey that has inspired us and driven us to seek the answers that have led to the information in this book. We sincerely trust that this book brings you not only the answers you're seeking but also provides peace and comfort. Most of all, that this book delivers the HOPE needed to fight back and WIN!

CONTENTS

DISCLAIMER

This information represents the views of the writers. These opinions are based on their interpretations of studies published in medical journals as well as their professional experiences. These opinions do not represent the views of the Yale-New Haven Hospital, Yale University or the Department of Veteran's Affairs.

The treatment information in this book is not intended as medical advice to replace the expertise, judgment and direction of your cancer care team. It is designed to help you and your families make informed decisions together with your doctor.

Your doctor may have reasons for suggesting a treatment plan different from these treatment options. Don't hesitate to ask him or her questions about your treatment options.

For more information:

American Cancer Society at 800-227-2345 or visit www.cancer.org.

A NOTE TO THE READER

Dr. Narayan: As a physician I have seen thousands of patients with melanoma, and I am continually struck by how often they have the same questions, fears, and misconceptions. What magnified their fears and concern was the fact there was not a single source to which I could direct them.

Another common need is a resource that would help support, not just the physical needs of treating melanomas, but also the non-medical needs of patients and caregivers. This resource is a holistic guide that also addresses the issues of physical well-being, diet, exercise and spiritual well-being.

By no means is this a comprehensive textbook for the care of a melanoma patient or survivor. It is intended to be a user-friendly book and a guide that offers information and hope to melanoma patients, their families, friends, and anyone who is genuinely concerned with the most serious of skin cancers.

About the Expert: Dr. Deepak Narayan

Deepak Narayan is a Professor of Surgery and a Surgical Oncologist at Yale who specializes in the treatment of melanomas and skin cancers. He has pioneered new reconstructive techniques for cancer and has over 100 publications in peer-reviewed journals.

Dr. Narayan has an active research interest in melanomas and is a co-investigator in the prestigious NIH-funded SPORE (Special Program of Research Excellence) Grant.

He is currently the Chief of Plastic Surgery at the West Haven Veterans Administration Hospital.

As a melanoma surgeon with extensive experience, Dr. Narayan provides patients with a unique resource of treating melanomas as well as reconstructing the defects that can occur from melanoma surgery.

He is an expert in specialized procedures for melanoma treatment and has won numerous awards for research, teaching, and clinical excellence. Dr. Narayan has been continually listed in *America's Top Surgeons* since 2002 and *The Best Doctors in America* since 2007, as well as Castle Connolly's, *Top Doctors*.

He has received the following awards for his research: American Cancer Society, Basic Oncology Research Award 1995, Swebilius Cancer Research Award American Society of Maxillofacial Surgeons Research Award 1998.

Please visit: www.yalesurgery.org/plastics/surgeons/narayan.aspx, to contact Dr. Narayan.

About the Expert: Lisa Lynn

Lisa Lynn has devoted 25 years of her career and practice to the fields of health and wellness personal training and coaching, specializing in metabolic weight loss and performance nutrition, as well as spiritual mentorship.

She is best known for her 13 years as Martha Stewart's personal trainer who has said, "Lisa is the only trainer that made a difference."

Lynn is also a regular go-to nutrition and fitness expert on The Dr. Oz Show, appearing in two of his highest rated episodes. Many major media outlets frequently use Lynn to provide feedback and direction in various segments showcasing her expertise.

Lynn has vast experience in the field of fitness and nutrition. Additionally, she has earned six Educational Certificates from the International Sports and Sciences Association's Professional Division including Certified Fitness Trainer, Specialist in Performance Nutrition, Fitness Therapy, and Elite Trainer.

Lynn's years of research in metabolic boosting and performance nutrition resulted in the development of her LynFit Leaner Lifestyle Series, specially designed to promote healthy fat loss by boosting the most sluggish and stubborn metabolisms.

Along with being a busy mom and wife, she maintains a diverse portfolio of clients including professional bodybuilders, actors, CEO's and real-world people from across the country.

How to Use this Book

So you just found out you have a melanoma. Perhaps your dermatologist cut out a mole and called you with a diagnosis or your primary care doctor scraped out a spot, which, to everyone's surprise, turned out to be a melanoma.

If you are confused, terrified, paralyzed by the diagnosis about what to expect, what the treatment will be or whether you will live or die, then please continue reading.

This book does not tell you everything written about melanomas. It does tell you what you do need to know and can be your guide as you navigate this difficult time and diagnosis. This book is meant to help empower you in your battle against melanoma because knowledge is power.

You don't need to read all the chapters in this book. Reading the introductory chapter gives you a great handle on everything else in the book, and we very strongly urge you to spend some time going through at least that chapter.

This book is divided into **three** major parts.

The **first part** deals with the basics of what melanoma is and how you can effect changes in your lifestyle to diminish your chances of getting a melanoma. The part we have the most control over is exposure to the sun and ultraviolet rays. Therefore, this is the largest part of this section.

The **second part** deals with the diagnosis and treatment of melanoma. The chart that you see on page 43 is important. We strongly urge you to spend a few minutes looking at it. It is quite simple to understand and summarizes the entire range of treatment from soup to nuts and gives you a birds-eye view of what to expect in every major scenario.

The **third part** focuses on wellness (physical as well spiritual), and how to be a thriver rather than a survivor. Studies suggest that patients who combine all aspects: the physical, mental and spiritual, heal faster, with some having even survived a hopeless prognosis.

Cancer is a scary diagnosis, but there is more hope than you think. No matter what situation you're facing, this book will bring you hope, and let you know that you're not alone.

This book will provide you with the resources to not only become your personal melanoma detective but also arm you with information needed to overcome it.

Knowing the most important features of your disease will help you to participate in the treatment, ask the appropriate questions of your physicians, calm your anxiety about the unknown, and stomp out the melanoma. The more you know about melanoma, the more you can be your own health advocate. You will feel empowered to make the choices that are right for you when it comes to the care, treatment plan, and management of this disease.

It doesn't matter who you are or where you live; you can use this book as a guide to help yourself understand melanoma and begin the healing process.

So take a deep breath, think pleasant thoughts and let's get started.

INTRODUCTION: DR. NARAYAN

In the United States alone, most people are of the mindset that melanoma is just another skin cancer. Not true. Nearly 60,000 Americans will be diagnosed this year, of which 8,000 will die.

Who else is living with melanoma?

- A 46-year-old health and fitness expert who noticed she had a mole on her leg that was changing.
- An otherwise healthy 8-year-old girl who had a pink lump on her chest.
- A 65-year-old, healthy successful businessman planning retirement, with a brown patch on his cheek.
- A 75-year-old African-American doctor with a black discoloration under his thumbnail.

These patients are good examples of how deceptive and varied a melanoma diagnosis can be.

Melanoma has no boundaries and can affect the most unsuspecting people. Melanoma can pop up anywhere, on anyone, at any time. Its lack of symptoms makes it a challenging disease to find and treat.

I've treated thousands of patients in the last 15 years. Unfortunately, I expect to see many more because the number of melanoma cases is rising at a rate faster than any other cancer. Melanoma can strike any age, gender, and socio-economic group. It is quickly becoming one of the most familiar cancers among the general population.

Sadly, melanoma has become the most common cancer among women aged 25–29. Among women aged 30–34, it is second only to lung cancer, which is the leading cancer in both men and women.

With such a dramatic increase in the incidence of melanoma, it's more important than ever before to educate and empower ourselves with the basic understanding of malignant melanoma. What it is, how it's diagnosed and treated, and what you can do to protect yourself from this deadly form of skin cancer.

As a Melanoma Specialist (practicing board certified physician) and clinical researcher, I'm in a unique position because I am involved with the latest cutting edge treatments that could potentially save your life.

The good news is that, with early detection, melanoma has a high cure rate. However, there is controversy when it comes to how to treat melanoma in its later stages. The survival rate for patients with metastatic melanoma continues to be 15–20 percent over 10 years despite the amount of research that's been done. We experts don't always agree on the best course of action.

It's little wonder then why patients are so confused and afraid. The fact that melanoma can strike healthy individuals in the prime of their lives can be scary. Most of us are not prepared or equipped for the medical or psychological issues we will be forced to face when confronted with melanoma.

I've learned through the years that most melanoma patients are scared, not to mention overwhelmed when faced with their diagnosis. They also have many questions that need to be answered.

The treatment of malignant melanoma requires the cooperation of many types of doctors with expertise in a variety of areas such as dermatology, surgery, oncology, radiation oncology, diagnostic radiology and pathology. I am privileged to work at Yale University and the flagship Yale-New Haven Hospital, with colleagues from various specialties who are at the forefront of the most cutting edge research. They are in fields as wide ranging as molecular biology, genetics, immunology (which is revolutionizing our particular approach to the care and treatment of malignant melanoma), Medical Oncology, Dermatology, and Radiation Therapy.

At Yale, we have established a team approach to the diagnosis and treatment of malignant melanoma—the so-called Tumor Board. By treating patients with the team approach (which includes everyone from basic scientists, clinical practitioners and nursing specialists, social workers, geneticists, and psychologists) we aim to provide the most comprehensive care for our patients. We deal with their physical needs as well as the emotional challenges they face, which we find critical to their healing.

This book will aim to provide you with this same information, so no matter where you live, you can receive the help you need to battle this deadly disease and WIN THE FIGHT against melanoma.

Thanks to research, change is happening at a rapid pace. It will be increasingly important for patients and their physicians to obtain the most up-to-date information to make the best medical decisions.

It's impossible to mention every single variable this disease presents. Patients need to work closely with their doctors, to better understand medical terms, and to provide insight into why we choose one particular procedure over another or one test over another.

A Patient's Perspective: Lisa Lynn

My Melanoma Miracle

The doctor said, "I've got bad news and good news." Words that immediately strike fear into your heart, because once you hear *bad news* you quickly tune out anything else that is said. These were words that I had never imagined hearing. Words that, even though they were not a part of my plan, were spoken to me regarding a disease that is no respecter of persons. I refuse to call it the big C. It will not be my master. I avoid doctors at all cost, as I tend not to trust them. They make a big deal out of everything, and honestly, this motivates me to stay fit and healthy.

You know that inner voice we all have that speaks to us when we just know something is wrong? I felt an *urge from above* (if you will), and finally got the courage to ask the doctor to remove a troublesome mole. He said, "You're worrying too much. We've been watching it and measuring it, and it's okay—really." I said, "No, I want it off now. I'm a busy mom, and I need to get it out of the way."

If I had not listened to that inner voice that I call God's little nudge, I might not be here today. I was floored when the results came back, and the doctor uttered those words I had never thought I would hear: "The bad news, it's melanoma. The good news is that you caught it early."

To be honest, it didn't register at first. I assumed it was one of those basic calls that we can all expect at some time or another. Then I went home, searched Google and read, *the deadliest form of skin cancer*. Most people are of the mindset that melanoma is *just skin cancer*. Not true. Over 60,000 Americans will be diagnosed this year, and 8,000 will die. In the United States, one person dies each hour, every day, from melanoma. It is the number one killer of women aged 25–29.

None of us ever wants to hear these words come out of our doctor's mouth, "I have bad news, you've got cancer." Even if it's followed with, "the good news is, we caught it early." You are still *marked by the beast* forever, and if you have ever been told that you have cancer, you know the terror you live with every day of your life. Every headache makes you think it's brain metastasis. Every time you get a simple cold you think it's a sign *the beast* is back, and you live every day of your life praying that a cure is discovered.

I was scared and immediately shut down, both physically and emotionally. I felt shame, guilt and anger, feeling that my body had let me down. I'm a fitness and nutrition expert; how could my body, which I take such good care of, let me down this way? Then I slipped into denial and put the appointment to the surgical oncologist off. I just wanted this problem to go away. The worst part was I didn't want to tell anyone—not even my closest friends who could offer me support. I suffered in my silent screaming hell.

What I didn't know at the time was that my faith was being upgraded and that being on the receiving end of this life-threatening illness would give my life a whole new meaning. I vowed only one outcome, to WIN THIS FIGHT. There was no other option.

It made me realize how vulnerable we all are every day. Vulnerability, my least favorite emotion. I heard a whisper in my ear that this was another opportunity. At that moment, I got off my *pity-potty* as my life was flashing before my eyes. I decided that I GET TO CHOOSE HOW I RE-SPOND TO CIRCUMSTANCES and that CANCER DOES NOT DEFINE ME, OR WHO I AM.

Cancer has taught me how to live life to the fullest and to never waste one single day worrying, or not letting the people I know how very important they are to me. I decided that I would use this battle with cancer as a way to inspire and educate others, to reach and empower as many people as I can to fight back and embrace this challenge. Cancer doesn't get to decide.

.

Everything happens for a reason. I'm on a mission to help you get stronger physically, mentally and spiritually so you too can WIN THE FIGHT and STOMP OUT melanoma. This book will take you beyond surviving and teach you how to thrive even in the worst possible scenarios. It's our attitude that causes us to thrive in anything, and *we get to choose*.

Stay Strong,
Lisa Lynn
Melanoma Survivor and Thriver

P.S. Remember: Google is not God

DID YOU KNOW?

We all have cancer cells in our body, but not all of us will develop cancer.

Why does cancer strike one person yet pass by another? While we can't control everything in our life, we get to decide how to fight back. While we can't control the environment or what we're exposed to on a daily basis, we have more control than we think. We can give cancer a run for its money by being the kind of person cancer doesn't like. How do you become that kind of person? That's what this book will teach you—How to "WIN THE FIGHT" and STOMP OUT CANCER!

WIN THE FIGHT

STOMP OUT MELANOMA

THE BASICS

ONE

WHAT IS CANCER?

If you or a loved one has been diagnosed with melanoma, you're most likely full of questions and feelings of anxiety and confusion. I'm sure you are wondering what it all means. What's the difference between melanoma compared to other skin cancers? The big question, of course—how serious is it? The precise answers provided in this book will help you begin to recover and heal. We tried to answer these questions as simply as possible, yet we wanted to provide you with the most thorough information to arm you with the knowledge needed to Win the Fight. Knowledge is power.

Our bodies are made up of hundreds of millions of living cells. The normal healthy cells in our body grow, divide, and die in an orderly fashion continuously, which is essential for replacing old worn out cells. The surface of your skin is a good example. When we are young, normal cells divide faster. That allows us to grow. In adulthood, most cells divide only to replace the worn-out or dying cells to aid in repairing injuries.

Cancer begins when the cells in a part of our body start to grow out of control. There are many different kinds of cancer, but they all start the same way—out of control growth of abnormal cells. Cancer cell growth is different from normal cell growth. Instead of dying, these unhealthy cells continue to grow and form new abnormal, unhealthy cells. There needs to be a healthy critical balance of cell growth and division. This balance is regulated by our genes, which are made up of our DNA. If our DNA is damaged, the cells life cycle can become altered, and begin to divide out of control. This uncontrolled division is how and why tumors (tumor means mass or swelling) are created and formed. The bottom line is that healthy cells become cancer cells because of DNA change and damage.

The unique ability that allows them to grow out of control and invade other healthy tissues is what makes a cell a "cancer cell".

I'm sure you're asking, "What causes our DNA to change or mutate?" People can inherit damaged DNA, that is they are born with a DNA flaw. A mutation is an error in the chemical code of a gene. Most DNA change/damage is caused by a misreading of the code that happens while the normal cell is reproducing, or by something in the environment. As a result, the protein produced

1

by the gene is flawed and cannot perform its normal function. These dangerous or malfunctioning proteins can lead to cancer.

While there are many reasons DNA mutates (including the hereditary factors discussed earlier), the ones we will focus on are the factors you have control over. Factors like cigarette smoking and exposure to radiation and ultraviolet light such as the sun, and the most lethal, tanning beds/booths. The latest research shows that viruses may also cause our DNA to mutate. Whatever the cause of the DNA mutation, if the cells continue to divide without stopping, eventually cancer cells form a tumor or growth. When this process happens in our skin cells, it's called skin cancer. There are some cancers that don't form tumors, leukemia being one of them. Instead, these cancer cells invade the blood and blood-forming organs, and they circulate through other tissues, where they grow.

It doesn't pay to worry about the things you can't change, but it always pays off to change the things that are in your control. As they say, "an ounce of prevention is worth a pound of cure."

WHY IS IT SERIOUS?

Cancer cells often travel to other parts of the body, where they begin to grow and form new tumors that replace the normal healthy tissue. This process is called metastasis. Metastasis happens when the cancer cells get into the bloodstream or lymph vessels of the body. The severity of the disease/cancer is also determined by the size and speed of spread of the metastasis. These metastases can kill the patient because they can reach areas of the body that cannot be cut out, such as the brain. They can spread to so many organs that they cannot be removed or treated adequately with medications or surgery.

So what exactly is a tumor? A tumor just refers to a growth that produces a lump or a swelling. A tumor does not always mean that it is cancerous. A tumor that is aggressive in its growth and spread is called malignant. This is another word for cancer.

Tumors that remain small and don't spread are called benign, and most times are less threatening. Benign tumors aren't so innocent as they can cause problems by growing very large, pressing on other organs and tissues. However, benign tumors cannot invade the healthy tissue the way malignant (cancerous) tumors can. Since benign tumors cannot metastasize or spread to other parts of the body, these tumors are almost never life threatening, and easier to treat, than malignancies or cancers.

No matter where cancer may metastasize (spread), it's always named after the place where it started. For example, breast cancer that has spread to the liver is still called breast cancer metastatic to the liver, not liver cancer. Similarly when a melanoma spreads to the lungs, it is called melanoma metastatic to the lung, not lung cancer. This is a common cause of confusion among patients.

Each type of cancer behaves differently and has its own personality. For instance, melanoma and breast cancer are very different diseases. They grow at different rates and respond to different treatments.

That's why it's important to talk to your doctor about your treatment concerns and not rely on the Internet for facts.

DID YOU KNOW?

Most patients get treatment advice from their friends or the Internet vs. their doctor or medical team. This is important, as melanoma is treated very differently than other cancers. Oftentimes, well-meaning friends may confuse us more, which can create unnecessary stress. You need to stay focused on the specific treatment that is aimed at your particular kind of cancer for the best results.

WHAT IS MELANOMA?

Melanoma is cancer that starts in a particular type of skin cell called a melanocyte. A melanocyte is a specific type of skin cell that has pigment or a colored protein that gives it its distinctive character. When these cells change as a result of inherited DNA damage or environmental reasons such as ultraviolet rays, a melanoma can occur.

A melanoma is a malignant (cancerous) tumor of the skin cells called melanocytes. It's also called malignant melanoma and cutaneous melanoma.

WHAT'S THE DIFFERENCE BETWEEN MELANOMA VS. OTHER TYPES OF SKIN CANCERS?

It's helpful to know the normal structure and function of healthy skin to grasp what makes melanoma so different. We will make a brief detour to explain the various parts of the skin and then go on to the other skin cancers. If you are familiar with this, you can skip to the next section.

SKIN 101

The skin is the largest and one of the most complex organs in your body. It's also one of the most vulnerable because it's the most exposed organ.

Can you imagine what life would be like without our skin? The skin is made up of three layers: epidermis (closest to skin), dermis (which is the larger, inner layer of the skin), and sub cutis (which is the deepest layer of skin). Each layer has an important job and contains highly specialized skin cells arranged in sub-layers.

The top layer of the skin, called the epidermis, is very thin and yet has a significant function. It protects the deeper layers of skin and organs of the body from the harshness of the environment. Knowing this, you can understand why we need to protect it by avoiding the sun, nourish it with healthy food and keep it hydrated by drinking lots of water. Everyone seems to forget to be picky about what we put on our skin as far as lotions and creams are concerned. Our skin absorbs most anything it comes into contact with, and many of these things can be toxic, including sunscreens.

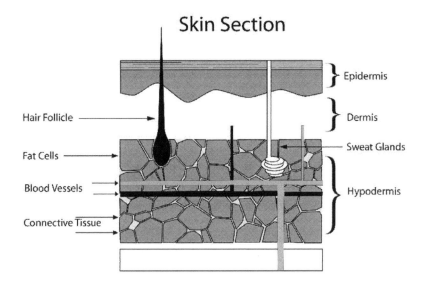

The Epidermis
The Epidermis contains three other layers:

The top or outer layer, which is called stratum corneum, is made of dead cells because these cells do not divide but continually slough off, and completely renew every 25–50 days. The cells in this layer are called squamous cells because of their flat shape.

Below that is the basal layer or the inner layer of the epidermis. The cells of the basal layer are called basal cells, which continuously divide to form new keratinocytes. These new keratinocytes replace the older keratinocyte cells as they slough off the skin's surface.

Intertwined in this layer is where the melanoma action occurs and is where the melanocytes, the cells that become melanoma, are found. These cells make the brown pigment called melanin, which makes the skin brown or tan. Melanin isn't bad and serves a purpose. It protects the deeper layers of skin from the harmful effects of the sun and ultraviolet radiation. The tan we refer to as "healthy glow" is an indicator of skin damage. As your skin gets darker, it means it needs more protection. Looking at it in a scientific way makes a tan seem unappealing and not quite as pretty doesn't it?

The Dermis
The middle layer of skin is called the dermis. The dermis is much thicker than the epidermis. It contains hair follicles, sweat glands, blood vessels, and nerves that are held in place by collagen. Collagen is made by cells that are called fibroblasts. Collagen is not only the secret to keeping your skin looking healthy, but it also gives skin its resilience and strength.

Collagen is another reason to eat healthy, as we need nourishing food for our body to perform these amazing processes.

Subcutis
The deepest layer of the skin is called the subcutis. It's also the lowest part of the skin/dermis, and it forms a network of collagen and fat cells. The subcutis helps our bodies conserve heat and has a shock absorbing effect that protects our organs from injury.

Our skin is the most vital organ of our body. It protects all other organs that keep us alive the same way a security guard protects precious assets. The skin is the ultimate defender when it comes to winning the fight. Protecting it is the best defense. When our skin changes color or gets tanned or burned, it's letting us know that damage has occurred. Our system is going off to warn us that harm is occurring the same way the alarms in our homes notify us when an intruder enters, allowing us to protect ourselves from danger. While sun damage isn't the only cause of melanoma, it's probably the most important reason We can do more to protect ourselves than we realize.

Under the epidermis, the deeper layers of the skin are separated from the basement membrane or the deepest layer of skin. This is an important structure because it serves as a significant barrier. When skin cancer becomes more advanced, it has grown through the basement membrane. Once it's reached this deep layer it passes by all of the other layers of skin such as the dermis (which contains hair follicles), sweat glands, and the blood vessels and nerves that are held in place by collagen. These give our skin its resilience and strength. Melanoma invading these deeper layers of skin is what makes it more severe than other forms of skin cancer, and is why it's known as the most deadly form of skin cancer.

The deeper layer of the skin, also known as the dermis, is where the blood vessels, the lymphatic vessels, and the nerves are found. The lymph vessels in this layer can pick up specialized cells, including melanoma cells, and carry them to the lymph nodes. From there, melanomas may travel through the lymphatic and vascular systems and can spread to almost any other part of the body. The melanoma cells may also directly invade the blood vessels elsewhere.

Healthy Skin Tip: The epidermis is made up of mostly keratinocyte cells, which make an essential protein called keratin. Keratin gives skin strength and flexibility and also makes the skin waterproof. A healthy diet is critical for maintaining healthy skin.

Now we can answer the question: What's the Difference Between Melanoma vs. the Other Types of Skin Cancers?

Non-Pigmented (Colored) Skin Cancers
Most common forms of skin cancer are of the non-pigmented type. Some examples of these are **basal cell carcinoma** and **squamous cell carcinoma**, which are named after the cells that caused them. While no skin cancer is a *good* cancer, these are fairly easy to cure, especially if they are caught early.

Believe it or not, **basal cell carcinoma** is *the most common human cancer* and accounts for 30 percent of all cancers in the United States. The most common places basal cell carcinomas are found are the parts of the body exposed to the sun, such as the face, nose, and ears, as well as the scalp. Basal cell can sometimes be trickier to identify because it looks rounder and is occasionally pigmented, so it's often confused with a melanoma. Either way it's always better to have a growth checked, to be safer than sorry.

Even though it's relatively common, basal cell carcinoma very rarely spreads to other parts of the body the way melanoma can. Treatment of basal cell carcinoma is still required since it can disrupt the surrounding healthy/normal tissues. Basal cell carcinomas on the nose, ear, and eyelid are often more prone to recurrence, so it's important to make sure they are completely removed, or treated. If you, or your loved one, have basal cell carcinoma, it's important to be examined at least yearly by a skilled dermatologist. The odds of recurrence are high, and chances are if you've had one basal cell, you'll most likely develop more.

Squamous cell carcinoma is the second most common skin cancer, and it occurs when the keratin producing cells in the skin divide out of control. It strikes 100,000 people each year in the United States. It's most likely to affect the people who have difficulty tanning and are prone to burn when exposed to the sun for a prolonged period. People with fair complexions, who burn easily and are freckled (particularly those of English, Scottish, Irish-Celtic and German descent) tend to have a higher risk/frequency.

Both basal cell and squamous cell carcinoma most commonly occur on sun-exposed parts of the body and interestingly are more common in men. However, squamous cell is the most dangerous of the two because it's more aggressive and grows more rapidly. This causes the destruction of the healthy tissues. It can also metastasize to other parts of the body.

That's why it's critical to have your skin regularly checked, especially if you spend lots of time in the sun or have been in tanning beds during your lifetime.

Squamous cell carcinomas appear on the skin as slightly raised nodules and can be reddish or even present as a sore that does not heal. These areas may grow over a period of weeks to months. The severity depends on their size, as well as how deep they are located within the layers of skin. Squamous cells that are missed and not caught early can spread locally, as they are given freedom to go deep into the skin.

The only way to tell the severity is to have it biopsied so the characteristics of the cells can be identified. When squamous cell carcinomas spread, they may send cells to the lymph nodes or nearby organs.

> **Despite the title above, it's not true that all basal cell or squamous cell cancers do not have color or pigments. A few of them actually do have color. Similarly, not all melanomas have color. The non-colored melanomas, the so-called amelanotic melanomas, look like pink or orange nodules or lumps. That is why it's important to see your dermatologist regularly.**

It's important to have all lymph nodes all over your body checked. In aggressive cases, it may be necessary to have surrounding internal organs evaluated, as well as have a CT scan or CAT scan, which is nothing more than a special X-rays.

ARE THERE DIFFERENT TYPES OF MELANOMAS?
Yes. The most commonly recognized types are:

- Superficial spreading

- Nodular
- Acral lentiginous
- Lentigo maligna melanoma

There are rarer types such as the **desmoplastic** melanoma and the internal or **mucosal melanomas.**

Melanoma-in- situ (or MIS) refers to the earliest stage of a melanoma. Any of the four types can begin as an MIS. The cure rate for this stage is very close to 100 percent.

The superficial spreading type is the most common. It accounts for about 60 percent of all melanomas.

The nodular melanomas account for about 15–20 percent of all melanomas.

The Acral-lentiginous types, 5–10 percent, are usually seen in the hands or feet (palms, soles, nail beds) and are relatively more common in African Americans.

The lentigo maligna form, 5–10 percent, is usually seen on the face or areas that have intense sun exposure and damage and typically in the elderly.

All these melanomas have two types of growth patterns. They can spread into the skin—the so-called radial spread or radial growth phase, or deep into the tissue.

The vertical growth phase—when the melanoma grows into the deeper parts of the skin, is considered the more dangerous type of growth since it is associated with a greater chance of spread or metastasis.

KNOW YOUR MOLES!

It's helpful to learn the essential differences between a melanoma, harmless skin lesions, and other types of skin cancers. This might actually help you to better develop a sharp eye that can help you spot a melanoma. It's also important to keep a close watch on all of your moles because cancer can develop from almost any cell in or on the skin and in your body. Certain cells are more likely to become cancerous than others.

Go from melanoma to "Mela-No-More" by being able to distinguish the difference between a melanoma mole and a mole that's harmless.

MOLES THAT CAN CHANGE TO MELANOMA

You may hear your doctor call your mole a *nevus*. Nevi is the plural of nevus. A nevus just means a birthmark but nowadays is used to describe moles colored or otherwise.

A common nevus, or mole, is the typical mole that's been biopsied, and the pathologist has categorized it as such, because of where the growth is located in the layers of skin. A common nevus will occasionally develop unusual features that make it stand out from all of the others. These unusual moles are called atypical or dysplastic nevi and are different from common nevi in that they are more likely to form melanomas.

WHAT IS A NEVUS?

A nevus is a scientific term for a mole, or to use doctor-speak, a benign melanocytic tumor. Moles are not usually present at birth, but they begin to appear in childhood which is why some doctors might overlook these moles. Most of them will never cause any problems, but a person who has many moles is at a high risk of melanoma even if they were present at birth.

Dysplastic nevi may look a little like melanoma and also like an ordinary mole. They are often larger than other moles and have an abnormal shape or color. Dysplastic nevi can appear just about anywhere on the body. Areas that have been exposed to the sun as well as areas like the buttocks and scalp that have been covered. Only a small number of dysplastic nevi develop into melanomas, and most never become cancerous.

The lifetime melanoma risk may be 10 percent for those with many dysplastic nevi, a condition that is sometimes referred to as dysplastic nevus syndrome.

Dysplastic nevi often run in families. If you have dysplastic nevi and have a close relative who has had melanoma, your lifetime risk is elevated. If you have a large number of dysplastic nevi, and several close relatives who have had melanoma, your lifetime risk goes up 50 percent or more. People with dysplastic nevus syndrome should have periodic, thorough skin examinations performed by a skilled dermatologist. In some cases, full body photographs are taken to help the doctor recognize which moles are changing and growing. Many doctors recommend that people be taught to do monthly skin exams and become experts in sun protection.

Do you have fair skin, freckle easily and light hair? Your risk of melanoma is more than 10-times higher because skin pigment has a protective effect. Caucasians with red or blond hair or fair skin that burns or freckles easily are also at an increased risk. Red haired people have the highest risk of them all. If you have any of these risk factors, you can't be too safe when it comes to sun protection.

TYPES OF NEVUS

Dysplastic nevi are also sometimes called atypical nevi (yes, it is confusing). Atypical nevi are:

- Larger than 5 millimeters in diameter
- Have inconsistent coloration
- Irregular or notched edges
- Blurry or non-definitive borders
- Can be scaly or lumpy (however keep in mind these lesions can be smooth as well, so when in doubt, check it out)

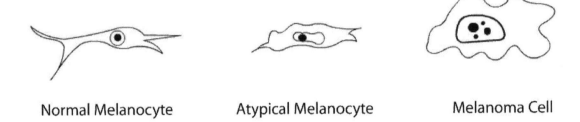

Normal Melanocyte   Atypical Melanocyte   Melanoma Cell

What makes atypical nevi different from common nevi is that they are more likely to develop into melanoma, and we still aren't sure why.

These atypical nevi are found in 5–10 percent of the population, but 30–40 percent of melanoma patients have atypical nevi, which suggest a high correlation. Of course, there are many people with atypical nevi/moles that do not develop melanoma.

> **As with all moles, (regardless of the various names given to them) if you notice any changes such as size, color or bleeding, these are not a good sign and you should have it checked out right away. In general, for all the moles described, anything larger than an eraser on a pencil or 6 millimeters should bear careful watching.**

You may encounter the following terms when you look at a pathology report or when the doctor tells you the results of your biopsy.

Types of Nevus (moles)

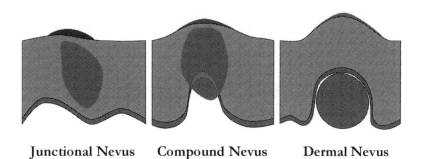

Junctional Nevus   **Compound Nevus**   **Dermal Nevus**

- Junctional Nevus: Occurs only in cells in the epidermis (non-vascular outer layer of skin)
- Compound Nevus: Contains cells in both the epidermis and the dermis, or both outer and deeper layer of skin
- Dermal Nevus: Cells are confined to the deeper layers and may not be pigmented since they are deeper
- Blue Nevus: A type of common nevus that's named "blue" because of its color, which is caused by melanin contained within the cells deep within the epidermis (outer layer of skin). These nevi are most common in women and can also occur on the scalp, hands, and feet. Most are considered benign lesions, yet surgical excision is usually recommended because melanoma can develop in this blue nevus.

DID YOU KNOW?

Cancers of other parts of the body, especially breast, lung and colon may spread to the skin? Be more vigilant if you have more than 50 moles, or 5 moles that are larger than 2 millimeters in diameter, as risk increases. Protect yourself by performing consistent and frequent skin checks weekly and see your doctor every 3 months.

Congenital melanocytic nevi are moles present at birth. The lifetime risk of developing melanoma with congenital melanocytic nevi is estimated at 0–5 percent depending on the size of the nevus. People with very large congenital nevi have a greater risk while the risk is much smaller for those with small nevi. Sometimes congenital nevi are removed by surgery so that they never become cancerous. Surgical removal of a congenital nevus is influenced by many factors, including its size, location and color. Many doctors recommend that a dermatologist examine congenital nevi regularly. People with congenital nevi should also be taught how to do monthly skin exams.

Having a single mole turn into cancer is very low, yet anyone with lots of large irregular moles has an increased risk of melanoma.

Congenital nevi that cover more than 5 percent of a child's body have much higher mortality risk, according to studies. Because of this risk, doctors advise the patient's family to have them removed.

A Spitz nevus is a kind of skin tumor that sometimes looks like melanoma. Sometimes doctors have trouble telling Spitz nevi from true melanomas, even when looking at them under a microscope. Most times they will be removed just to be safe. Most of these nevi are benign and do not spread. They are usually seen in children.

OTHER BENIGN TUMORS

Most tumors are benign, and these tumors that develop from other types of skin cells include the following:

- Seborrheic Keratosis: Tan, brown, or black raised spots with a wax-like texture or rough surface. These are often called age spots.
- Hemangiomas: Benign blood vessel growths often called cherry or strawberry spots or port wine stains. These are usually red.
- Lipomas: Soft growths of benign fat cells
- Warts: Rough surfaced growths caused by a virus

There are many more benign skin tumors that are not very common. Most of these tumors rarely, if ever, develop into cancers. It's best to have a better understanding of different skin cancers and the benign growths. You will develop a sharp eye for the bad moles and worry less about benign moles when you learn what makes them different.

KNOWLEDGE IS THE POWER

Dark Spot

Freckle	Nevus (mole)
normal cells more pigment normal number of cells	slightly abnormal cells usually normal amount of pigment increased number of cells

What's the difference between a freckle and a mole (nevus)? As you know from reading the basics, the cells in our body that contain pigment or give skin its color are called melanocytes. The melanocytes have a pigment called melanin inside them which are stored in little ball-like structures called melanosomes.

When a melanocyte or a group of melanocytes in an area has a much larger number of these melanosomes, you get a freckle.

DID YOU KNOW?

- Melanoma's cure rate is 85 percent if caught early. Even if melanoma is caught in the advanced stages treatments can be very successful.
- Just one indoor tanning session increases the chances of developing melanoma by 20 percent, and each additional session during the same year boosts the risk almost another 2 percent.
- Sustaining 5 or more sunburns in youth increases lifetime melanoma risk by 80 percent.

A nevus, on the other hand, is formed when there is an increase in the number of melanocytes in the area. The cells may be a little different in shape and size than normal. Thus, each melanocyte in a nevus may have the proper number of melanosomes inside them but because there are such a large number of them they look dark and form a nevus or a mole. Sometimes it can be difficult to tell the difference between the two.

MELANOMA STATISTICS YOU NEED TO KNOW

- Skin cancer is the most common of all cancers. Luckily, melanoma accounts for less than 5 percent of skin cancer cases but causes over two-thirds of the skin cancer deaths.
- The American Cancer Society estimates that 70,230 melanomas will be diagnosed this year. Melanoma rates have continuously increased for the last 30 years.
- Melanoma diagnoses have been increasing in young Caucasian women, as well as older Caucasian men.
- The lifetime risk of melanoma, when you've had sunburns, is 80 percent, without any other risk factors.
- Melanoma, unlike many other cancers, has one of the widest age ranges. It occurs in younger and older people.
- Melanoma rates increase with age.
- Melanoma attacks people under 30-years-old and is even more frequent among teens that should be at their healthiest, but because of tanning bed use, melanoma is attacking our youth at a devastating rate.
- An estimated 9,940 people in the United States will die from melanoma in the year 2015, according to the American Cancer Institute.

MELANOMA FACTS

➢ Melanoma likes to strike Caucasians of European descent, especially if you are Celtic descent (Irish and Scottish).

➢ Melanoma can strike families. Ten percent of all melanoma cases are genetic.

➢ Melanoma loves young white females between 15 to 39-years-old who tan.

➢ Melanoma likes light eyes. The lighter your eyes, the larger your risk.

➢ Melanoma prefers light skin over dark skin, especially skin that burns easily and freckles.

➢ Melanoma is 10-times more common in Caucasians vs. African Americans.

➢ More moles equal higher melanoma risk.

➢ People with more than 50 atypical moles, or a family history of melanoma, are at an increased risk of developing melanoma.

➢ African American and Hispanics also get melanoma.

TWO

PREVENTION

WHAT IS A RISK FACTOR?

A risk factor is anything that affects your chance of getting cancer. Every cancer has its set of risk factors. A good example is smoking. Smoking is a risk factor for cancers of the lungs, mouth, larynx (voice box), bladder, kidney, and several other organs. We would run out of space if we listed them all.

While risk factors are important to note, they don't tell us everything. If you have a risk factor or several risk factors, it still does not mean you will get the disease. On the flip side, people who don't have any risk factors can develop melanoma. Scientists believe that several risk factors place you at a higher risk for melanoma, and you need to be aware of them to protect yourself. The following list of risk factors is by the level of importance.

Note: *This list only names the most common risk factors and does not cover all of them. Talk to your doctor for more information regarding your specific risk factors.*

Five factors that raise your risk of skin cancer:

Risk Factor One: You have a family history
If your mother, father, siblings, or children have had a melanoma, your risk is 50 percent greater than the average person.

Risk Factor Two: You have had a sunburn
Just one sunburn in childhood or adolescence more than doubles your chances of developing melanoma later in life. Even five mild sunburns over the course of your life can also double your risk.

Risk Factor Three: You have used a tanning bed

Indoor tanners, both past and present, are 74 percent more likely to develop melanoma than those who have never used a tanning bed. They also have a 69 percent increased risk for early-onset basal cell carcinoma.

Risk Factor Four: If you have fair skin and light-colored eyes

Pale women have less melanin—the skin's natural protection. Those with baby blue or green eyes are also more prone to skin cancer, especially ocular and eyelid melanoma, than women with deep brown irises.

Risk Factor Five: You live in a sunny or high-altitude area

Tropical climates expose you to strong UV radiation year-round. As for altitude, for every 1,000 feet above sea level you are, you increase your UV radiation exposure by 4–5 percent.

Let's go through this step by step:

RISK FACTOR ONE

Does Your Family Have A Melanoma History? If you have had a first-degree relative (mother, father, brother, sister or child) who has had melanoma, your risk is greater. Approximately 10 percent of all people with melanoma have a family history of the disease. Some of the increased risk may be due to a similar lifestyle of frequent sun exposure, a tendency toward fair skin, or a combination of both factors. It can also be caused by inherited gene changes or mutations. Gene mutations have been known to cause 10–40 percent of melanoma within families.

One of the first questions people ask is, "Should I get tested for the melanoma gene/s?"

This is known as the *Angelina Effect*. Since May 2013, when actress Angelina Jolie announced that she had a double mastectomy to lower her risk of breast cancer, doctors have seen an enormous jump in the number of genetic testing being done for breast cancer.

While Jolie had good reason to be tested, the United States Preventative Services Task Force doesn't recommend it because most of us don't have the genes that make a big difference in risk. Not only that, you can test negative, meaning you don't have the gene and can still get melanoma. Good genes can be damaged by overexposure to the sun, and bad genes don't always mean you'll get the disease.

Should you be tested anyway? We very strongly advise you to seek the help of a professional who deals with these issues—a Genetic Counselor.

The CDC's website can help you decide: www.cdc.gov/. Genetics isn't a guarantee. It just means you're more susceptible. If you are genetically predisposed to melanoma, you should be even more religious about the lifestyle you lead to take every precaution possible so you can avoid melanoma.

The bottom line is bad genes don't mean you'll always get it, and good genes don't mean you won't.

What Kind Of Gene Are They Looking For? It's not the genes themselves we are worried about but whether or not they mutated. Genetic tests look for a mutation in the CDKN2A gene that accounts for about 35–40 percent of melanoma cases that run in families, according to www.cancer.gov. They are damaged versions of the genes that prevent the growth of abnormal cells.

Are There Any Other Genetic Susceptibility Variants That Increase The Risk Of Getting Melanoma? Yes. These variants are not the same as mutations. These variants are normal and appear to regulate how cells change as we grow and develop. The variants control when the gene switch gets turned on and off, in which organs, and at what time of life.

Most experts at this time do not suggest genetic testing for susceptibility variants, even if your family is at an increased risk, due to the genetic changes that our lifestyle may cause. We just don't understand enough about these variants to give sound advice to patients.

Even if you have great genes, a less than the optimal lifestyle filled with smoking and sunbathing can cause enough damage that can affect even the best genes. Just because you have bad genes doesn't mean you'll get melanoma.

It is suggested that you:

- Have regular skin exams by a skilled dermatologist
- Thoroughly examine your skin weekly, or at the very least, monthly

What's Your Personal History? If you've already had melanoma, your risk is increased 5–10 percent. People who have had melanoma have a small but definite chance that they can develop it again at some point in a brand new place. This means that melanoma does not come back, but an entirely new melanoma develops from scratch.

RISK FACTOR TWO
Ultra Violet Radiation Exposure—Exposure to ultraviolet (UV) radiation is the #1 risk factor for most melanomas. Sunlight is the primary source of UV radiation because it damages the DNA/genes in your skin cells. Tanning beds and booths are also sources of UV radiation.

This is how melanoma is attacking young girls who just want to look better in their prom dress or on the beach. People with high levels of exposure to radiation are at an elevated risk as well, and many of these UV sources are unsuspecting, such as phototherapy (used to treat psoriasis) and black light lamps.

A single sunburn can increase your chance of getting a melanoma. Ultraviolet rays play such an important role in the problem that we have a separate chapter for it.

The "TANOREXIA" Factor—the "Healthy Glow" That Kills Young Women

Skin cancer kills, but we continue to use these indoor tanning beds. Tanning beds might as well be coffins. Dermatologists now believe they are to blame for the alarming spike among young women in lethal melanoma cases. Melanoma is the second most common cancer in adults under 30-years-old. The problem is that women think that indoor tanning is a harmless way to get tan. Even worse, it's become a big part of their beauty routine year round.

According to researchers, melanoma rates have increased ten-fold among women ages 18–39 since 1970. In fact, melanoma is the new epidemic in young women. Of course, the usual suspects are partly to blame for the rise in deadly melanoma among women 20–30-years-old. The disappearing ozone layer adds to the fact that we are still getting sunburns even though we know better. Using tanning beds is chief among them. These numbers are alarming. According to the Centers for Disease Control and Prevention, 32 percent of Caucasian women ages 18–21 and 30 percent of Caucasian women ages 20–25 say they use indoor tanning beds.

RISK FACTOR THREE
Are You Addicted to a Tan? Even with all of the knowledge we have about the dangers of indoor tanning, young people continue to do it. Research shows that tanning is as addictive as some drugs. What makes this tanorexia addiction so hard to treat is that it's socially acceptable. Doctors are reporting that they are treating skin cancer patients who had tanned, get diagnosed with a basal cell carcinoma or melanoma, yet continue to tan. That's a powerful addiction. It's reminiscent of smokers who continue to smoke after a diagnosis of cancer. Tanners also report that they need the mood boost, and scientists can vouch for this. In fact, researchers report that tanning affects the part of our brain that is associated with reward. This is the kind of brain activity that keeps us coming back for more, and we get hooked.

The goal is to change the behavior of young women (or everyone for that matter) and get them to stop tanning so the incidence of melanoma will change. But how do we do this when women are in denial about how dangerous tanning beds are? Or worse, they become addicted to tanning because UV light has been shown to increase the release of opioid-like endorphins; feel-good chemicals that relieve pain, and generate feelings of well-being.

Take this quiz to find out if you have tanorexia:

- Do you continue to sunbathe even though you know the risk?
- Have your friends or family voiced their concern that you're always tan or are tanning?
- Do you stay tan year round?
- Do your tan lines take more time to fade?
- Have you avoided skin checks because you'd rather tan?
- Have you had skin cancer already, yet continue to tan?

If you answered "yes" to even one of these questions, we urge you to seek help from a qualified professional. It's possible you're suffering from tanorexia. Help and hope are available. Your life depends on it.

The best way to effect this change is to improve the social environment and remove the stigma associated with being pale.

The Wrong Message. One of the reasons young women are still tanning, despite health warnings, is the warnings of the dangers of indoor tanning are not only ineffective, but they are also deceptive. Thus, causing young people to have the attitude, "it will never happen to me, and if it does, I'll deal with it."

What about the delusion factor? Behavioral scientists at Sloan-Kettering Cancer Center in New York City surveyed more than 500 college students in the United States. Fifty-nine percent of indoor tanners say it's because, "everything causes cancer these days." Fifty-four percent said tanning beds are, "no more risky than lots of other things people do."

This defeatist attitude is killing young people that might otherwise live long healthy lives. They allow the tan benefits to win vs. making wise choices. It's critical that we spread the word that tans can kill. Indoor tanning is not a safe way to tan, and will not prevent or protect you from sunburns by giving you a base tan. In fact, nothing could be further from the truth. Getting tan is a sign that damage is already occurring to your skin. You need to know it's not only aging it, but this damage is happening on a deep cellular level. Tanning (UV exposure) damages healthy DNA. Good genes or not, you're destroying DNA every time you step into a tanning bed or stay in the sun longer than 15 minutes.

Pale Needs To Equal Pretty. The social pressure to be tan seems to be easing up. Stars like Nicole Kidman, Scarlet Johansen, Taylor Swift, Anne Hathaway; makeup gurus like Bobbi Brown, as well as all runway models, are paving the way when it comes to *pale is prettier*. In fact, most stars don't even get spray-tanned before a red carpet event anymore. Tanning is becoming passé. Many people agree that a tan is very "Jersey Shore-like", and pale is trending in high society women. The new understanding that is catching on is that remaining pale makes women look smarter and younger while tanning turbo-charges the aging process and causes wrinkles.

RISK FACTOR FOUR

Do you have fair skin and light-colored eyes? Pale women have less melanin, the skin's natural protection. Those with baby blue or green eyes are also more prone to skin cancer, especially ocular and eyelid melanoma, than women with deep brown irises.

RISK FACTOR FIVE

Do you live in a sunny or high-altitude area? During a plane trip, you are exposed to a higher level of UV rays. This puts pilots and crew who frequently travel in planes at an increased risk of melanoma.

Think you are healthy if you live in Denver? The reason there's more UV radiation in the so-called Mile High City is because it is exactly a mile above sea level, and there is the thinner air that accompanies high altitude. The sun has an easier time pushing through the thin mountain air, exposing Denverites to higher levels of a non-ionizing source of radiation: UV rays. This is true not just for Denverites but all high altitude. For every 300 meters, there is a 4 percent increase in UV exposure.

PREVENTION IS THE CURE!

Early detection and early treatment increase survival rates by about 98 percent according to www.cancer.net/cancer-types/melanoma/statistics. Ask any dermatologist and they will tell you— if you tan indoors, you're going to increase your risk for melanoma by 75 percent if you use a tanning bed before 35-years-old. In other words, there is a good chance you will become a statistic.

WHAT AREAS SHOULD YOU FOCUS ON?

Melanoma can be found anywhere on the skin but is most likely to be found on the chest and back (which are the most common sites in men). The legs are the most common site for women. The neck, face, and ears are also very common in both men and women. *Interestingly, melanoma can also develop on the palms of the hands, soles of the feet, and under the nails (which is more common in African Americans).* These areas represent more than half of all melanomas in African Americans, but fewer than 10 percent of melanomas show up in these areas in Caucasians. Having darkly pigmented skin might lower your risk factors, but isn't a guarantee that you will not get melanoma. Melanoma can develop anywhere on the body; such as eyes, mouth, and even the vagina.

WHO SHOULD BE WORRIED?

Melanoma is not particular and is found all over the world, in many nationalities. It is less prevalent among African Americans and very rare in Japan. Australia has the highest rate where melanoma affects 1 in every 60 Australians. Remember, knowledge, combined with action, is the best defense for you to become the person melanoma cannot attack.

WHAT'S AGE GOT TO DO WITH IT?

Unlike other cancers, melanoma is not as closely linked to aging. It is more likely to occur in older people yet melanoma rates are skyrocketing in younger people. It's important that you don't discount your risk because of your age. In fact, melanoma is one of the most common cancers in people younger than 30-years-old. If melanoma runs in your family, it can occur at any age. You can never be too safe.

GENDER BIAS

Melanoma has a gender bias. In the United States, men have a higher rate of melanoma than women. The majority of people diagnosed with melanoma are Caucasian men over 50-years-old. Adults over 40-years-old, especially men, have the highest annual exposure to UV. An estimated 43,890 new cases of invasive melanoma in men and 32,210 in women were diagnosed in the United States in 2014. Also, an estimated 6,470 men and 3,240 women in the United States died from melanoma in 2014, according to www.skincancer.org.

EXPOSED: THE RISK FACTORS YOU MAY NOT KNOW

Melanoma rates are skyrocketing and with good reason. Did you know that our current ozone layer (the ozone acts as a protective coating that shields out the harmful ultraviolet light) does not provide the same level of protection that it provided 30 years ago? Combine this lack of ozone protection with the popularity of sunbathing and love of outdoor activities and you've created the ideal conditions for melanoma.

We call this, the perfect melanoma storm.

If you love to golf, fish, water ski, garden, snow-ski, vacation in warm places at least once a year, have a second home on a lake or beach, or have a second or third getaway in a warm sunny place where you spend lots of time in the sun when your main hometown is cold and lacking sun— YOU ARE AT RISK.

I can hear you now, "Not me. We go north and snow-ski and snowmobile." Sound familiar? Guess what? Snow skiing is worse as the rays of the sun are amplified due to the reflection off the snow. Water skiing poses the same risk due to reflection.

Another high-risk situation is hiking. Hiking is most often done at high altitudes where sun and UV rays are the strongest therefore increasing exposure (also a *need to know* when you vacation or live close to the Equator). Most people don't think of these risk factors.

Before we move on, there is a growing concern over why young women are getting melanoma at alarmingly high rates. It's critical to look at the whole picture to see the cause and effect reasons.

THE MELANOMA-MOMMY FACTOR

Women tend to live a "mom and me" lifestyle as young moms. We spend our day taking our young children to the pool, beach or park. Bottom line, we take our precious kids outside for fun. This is especially alarming because most of the damage that causes melanoma happens when we are young. Just one blistering sunburn in childhood more than doubles a person's chances of developing melanoma later in life. According to one United States study, 54 percent of children become sunburned or tanned in their second summer versus 22 percent in their first.

"Children should not be getting sunburned at any age, especially since there is a range of very effective sun protection methods that can used," says Perry Robins, MD, President, The Skin Cancer Foundation. "Parents need to be extra vigilant about sun protection all the time." From ages 0–15 is when the melanoma groundwork is laid, not to mention the ultraviolet light accumulates for the rest of our lives. Think of it this way, each one of us has an ultraviolet budget, and every minute we spend outside between the hours of 9 a.m. to 3 p.m., we use this lifetime budget. We cannot erase or get it back. In fact, sunscreen provides a false sense of security for three reasons:

1. Sunscreens are not designed to block out the sun completely
2. We don't apply them correctly. A vast majority do not re-apply it as often as you are required to.
3. We don't use the right kind of sunscreen

Now think of your life. Is your young son or daughter in an outdoor sport like soccer, tennis or golf? Do they ski or horseback ride? How long are they outdoors and exposed to the sun on a daily basis? You can do the math; add up your sun exposure hours, and multiply them over 30 years, and you'll understand why melanoma strikes. Most people, when diagnosed with melanoma respond saying, "I'm never in the sun. I work 7 days a week." The sad part is, by the time of diagnosis, it's too late. The damage had been done before most of us turned 10-years-old.

SHOCKING SUN-TIME TEST

The next time you go outside, set the timer on your cell phone the second you step outside to see how much time you really spend outdoors.

UNUSUAL RISK FACTORS

Immune Suppression and Melanoma: If you've been treated with medicines that suppress your immune system, like steroids, your risk is increased. HIV is another cause of immune suppression, especially if it's not treated correctly.

Have You Had an Organ Transplant? You're at increased risks due to the drugs you need to take that suppress your immunity.

Lymphomas and Melanomas: If you have had lymphoma your risk of developing melanoma is higher, and the latest research indicates there may be a link.

Xeroderma Pigmentosum: This is a very rare disease where the DNA damage cannot be repaired by the body and can result in multiple melanomas.

WHAT SHOULD YOU BE LOOKING FOR? HOW TO SPOT A SUSPICIOUS MOLE

Self-skin checks are an early warning system. Did you know that patients find most melanomas, not a doctor? It helps if you know what to look for. If you spot a new dot that you suspect is melanoma, keep calm and carry on. Melanoma is easily treated when it's caught early.

Mark your moles and record them on your cell phone or a piece of paper. When using your cell phone be sure to use:

- Same light
- Same distance
- A tape measure

Mark the position of each mole, freckle, birthmark, bump, or scaly patch you see by making a dot on a body map.

- Draw a line from the dot and note the date, the size, and the color. Take a picture with your cell phone for best results.
- Check each mole for any change in size, color, or shape each time you perform your skin exam. Be sure to add the date and a brief description. (*Note: Some moles may have appeared since your last skin check, be sure to mark it and date it.*)
- Consistency and frequency are the best way to WIN this FIGHT. Stay on track by marking your skin checks each time you perform them, and enter your next skin check on your calendar. I enter mine in my Google calendar and set alerts as a reminder, so I don't forget.

FIVE WARNING SIGNS TO LOOK FOR

There are five primary warning signs of melanoma, the ABCDE's:
(http://melanoma.surgery.ucsf.edu/ | www.skincancer.org)

A - Stands for Asymmetry
If you drew a line through the center would each side match?

B - Stands for Border
Most melanomas have an irregular shape, with notched edges

C - Stands for Color
Melanomas are found in a variety of shades of brown or black, as well as some not so typical shades—a mix of red, white, and blue. Most moles are a uniform shade of brown.

D - Stands for Diameter
Most melanomas are larger than a ¼ inch (6 millimeters) in size, which is the size of a small pencil eraser. If you suspect, get it checked. The earlier you spot the melanoma, the smaller it is, the better.

E - Stands for Evolve Evolution or Change
Changes in your moles mean they are growing, and this is the most important thing to look for. It is imperative to keep a close watch for any moles or spots on the skin that change in shape, size or color. See your doctor right away if this happens. You should also be aware of any new or unusual sores, lumps, blemishes, markings or changes in your skin. Signs like crusty, scaly, oozing or bleeding skin as well as itchy, tender, painful skin could also be signs of skin cancer, or an early warning that it might occur.

Your doctor should check any spot on the skin that looks different from surrounding moles. Now is the best time to deal with it. Don't wait to call your doctor. If you are suspicious of a mark on your skin, call your doctor and let him know that you need to be seen right away.

THE SKIN SPECIALIST METHOD TO CHECK FOR POSSIBLE SIGNS OF MELANOMA

The ABCDE rule is helpful when it comes to detecting melanomas, but not all melanomas exhibit the ABCDE features. Specialists have another method they use. They look for the ugly duckling signs, and it's based on the fact that these melanomas look different (like ugly ducklings compared to other moles).

It's not always easy to tell the difference between a melanoma and an ordinary mole (even for doctors). It's important to show any suspicious mole to your doctor so they can use their specialized techniques, such as dermoscopy (also known as dermatoscopy epi luminescence microscopy [ELM], or surface microscopy), to look at suspicious spots on the skin more precisely. If you are a high risk, we strongly suggest that you see a skilled dermatologist who uses dermoscopy for maximum safety. You can ask when you book your appointment.

REMEMBER: THERE IS NO METHOD OF DIAGNOSING A MELANOMA WITH 100 PERCENT CERTAINTY, OTHER THAN A BIOPSY

THREE

Ultraviolet Rays, Sunscreens, UV Protective Clothing, Tanning Beds

The sun is truly the giver of life. So many natural processes are dependent on sunlight that it is little wonder that the sun has been worshiped by diverse communities all over the globe for thousands of years. However, this life-giving source also plays a significant role in the development of melanoma.

The rays of the sun contain waves of different levels of energy. The one that is relevant to this discussion are the ultraviolet rays. The UV rays are classified into three types based on a number called the wavelength of light that is measured in nanometers. A nanometer is one billionth of an inch.

Ultra Violet Radiation is Divided into Three Wavelength Ranges (Three Types):

1. UVA Rays (the same ones that make us tan) cause cells to age and cause damage to cell's DNA. They are linked to long-term skin damage (such as wrinkles), and they also play a role in some skin cancers. These rays can penetrate clouds and untreated glass.
2. UVB rays (the burning rays) can cause direct and immediate damage to the DNA and are thought to not only cause most sunburns but cause most skin cancers as well.
3. UVC rays are not a cause of skin cancer because they don't penetrate our atmosphere.

UVA and UVB rays only make up a small portion of the sun's wavelengths. They are the main culprit and cause of the sun's damaging effects on the skin. UVB rays are more lethal and cause most skin cancers, but we now know that there are no safe UV rays. Not only is the length of time spent exposed to UV radiation a concern, but it's also imperative that you understand that the intensity of the exposure matters just as much. If you are exposed to the sun for a shorter period, but the sun is strong, that's just as damaging. The bottom line is: If your skin is exposed for 15 minutes (which is considered a healthy dose) and you burn because the sun is strong that day, or you are near the Equator, it's just as damaging. This puts you at a higher risk.

The nature of the UV exposure also plays a role in melanoma development. Many melanomas are found on the legs, arms and trunk of the body from sunburns received as a child. Melanomas that develop on the hands, soles of the feet, underneath the nails, or internally (such as the mouth and vagina), are different from either of the other types of melanoma. They are not exposed to the effects of UV rays. Scientists believe that this group may be caused by other unknown factors.

> **ULTRAVIOLENT RADIATION EXPOSURE IS NOT THE SAME AS THE RADIATION EXPOSURE YOU GET FROM X-RAYS, AIRPORT SCANNERS OR ATOMIC EXPLOSIONS**

TAKE THE QUIZ

WHAT FITZPATRICK TYPE ARE YOU?
The Fitzpatrick Scale

Type I: Pale white, blond or red hair, blue eyes, freckles—Always burns, never tans

Type II: White, fair, blond or red hair, blue, green or hazel eyes—Usually burns, tans minimally

Type III: Cream white, fair with any hair or eye color—Sometimes mild burn, tans uniformly

Type IV: Moderate brown, typical Mediterranean skin tone—Rarely burns, always tans well

Type V: Dark brown, Middle Eastern skin types—Very rarely burns, tans very easily

Type VI: Deeply pigmented dark brown to black—Never burns, tans very easily

The Fitzpatrick Scale is an internationally recognized system of classifying skin types and risk for sunburn Types I, II and III. They are the most at risk for burns, and this is the group that must be religious about using sunscreen. It may not be possible to stay out of the sun altogether and indeed most people will rebel against it. What you can do, however, is to protect yourself against the harmful effects of the sun's rays by following the five necessary steps.

Ultraviolet Rays, Sunscreens, UV Protective Clothing, Tanning Beds

Five Tips for Safe Sun

1. Stay out of the sun during the peak UV ray time between 9 a.m. to 3 p.m. (or 10 a.m. to 4 p.m. according to some authorities)
2. Use sunscreen liberally (a shot glass full applied to all exposed parts of your body)
3. Re-apply it every 2 hours or sooner, if you are in the water (pool or sea)
4. If you must be outside at these times, seek the shade of an umbrella
5. Use a wide brim hat and protective glasses when you are out in the sun

Sun Screen and Sun Block

Sunscreens were initially developed for protection against UVB rays only.

There are two types of sunscreens. Sunscreens must contain ingredients that help prevent harmful radiation (the radiation for the UV range) from damaging the skin.

The first type is also called a sunblock. These are chemicals that physically bounce UV radiation with their particles like a shield. Titanium dioxide and zinc oxide are two FDA approved products in this category.

The second type, the so-called chemical sunscreens, contain compounds that absorb the UV rays without letting it harm the skin.

These are the different types you may see; Octinoxate, Oxybenzone, Octocrylene, and Avobenzone.

SPF stands for Sun Protection Factor, which is a laboratory test of a sunscreen's efficiency. It measures the amount of UV radiation needed to cause a burn on the protected skin as compared to the unprotected one.

What Sunscreen Should I Buy?

- Broad spectrum (blocks UVA and UVB rays)
- Water resistant, if you plan to be in the water. This used to be referred to as waterproof but was changed by the FDA to water resistant.
- Sunscreen with an SPF of 30 and higher. The FDA has recently forbidden the use of numbers above 50 in advertising for sunscreen. Anything and everything above 50 are now just called 50+. It is important to know that no matter how high the SPF, it does not necessarily mean one can stay longer in the sun. The reason is that there is no relationship between the percentage of SPF and the extent of protection. Beyond a certain point, the

higher numbers do not necessarily mean more protection. An SPF of 15, for example, can block out 94 percent of the harmful rays and an SPF of 30, up to 97 percent. An SPF of 60 percent could give you longer protection.

It is most important to remember that a sunscreen with twice the SPF does not mean one can stay out twice as long in the sun.

UV RAYS AND CLOTHES
Clothing can increase blocking of UV rays. Wet clothes are worse than dry ones in terms of blocking capacity. A tight weave is always better.

PROTECTIVE CLOTHING AND EYE WEAR
If you are going to go outside the simple truth is any cover is better than no cover. A simple tee shirt will do a better job than no tee shirt. Then why bother to invest in special UV protective clothes?

Regular clothes can block out UV rays but perhaps not as efficiently as specially designed ones. The UV protective clothing manufacturers utilize all the factors discussed. Also, they use special dyes that are engineered to disrupt and reflect UV light and offer a more consistent protection. They are useful for people with allergies to sunscreen or in children and adults who may forget to put on sunscreen at appropriate intervals or spend extended periods of time in the sun. These fabrics are specially designed to be breathable and can wick away moisture and dry quickly. For these reasons, they may actually feel cooler than regular tee shirts.

The type of clothing matters. In this case, polyester or nylon fares better than cotton or other natural fabrics in protection against UV rays.

Stretching the fabric opens up the weave and decreases the protective effect.

Optical Brighteners (the chemicals that make bright colors more vivid or those that keep whites whiter) found in some detergents can give the clothes laundered in them the capacity to block UV rays better than untreated materials. In fact, the more they are laundered in them, the better the protection. Rit Sun Guard™ laundry additive is available if you are the do-it-yourself kind of person.

UV RAYS AND CHILDREN
Our strong recommendation is that children under 6-months-old be kept in the shade rather than having sunscreen on them. If they have to be outside, parents should dress the children in hats

and protective clothing. Every child 6-months-old and over should always be covered with photoprotective clothing and sunscreen.

Like the SPF factor (sun protection factor), there is a rating for clothes called UPF. The difference in UPF and SPF is that UPF is a measure of blocking both UVA and UVB rays, while SPF measures block out UVB only. UPF stands for Ultra Violet Protection Factor.

UPF rating (Ultraviolet Protective Factor):

15–24	Good
25–39	Very Good
40–50	Excellent
50+	Most excellent

A rating of 50, for instance, means that the fabric will allow only 1/50th of available UV radiation to go through.

DRUGS, UV RAYS, AND THEIR INTERACTION

If you are taking medications, you must know that some drugs cause reactions in your skin when exposed to UV rays. These are called photosensitivity reactions and not everyone taking these drugs will have this problem.

There are two types of photosensitivity reactions. They are caused by different mechanisms in our body.

Phototoxic: This is the most common type of reaction. Phototoxic reactions result from a direct interaction of UV rays and the drugs in the skin. A few examples of drugs that can do this are painkillers (such as Ibuprofen, Aleve), antibiotics (such as Ciprofloxacin, levofloxacin, Bactrim tetracyclines), antifungals such as Griseofulvin, and anti-hypertensive drugs (such as Captopril, Verapamil, Amiodarone, Thiazides etc.).

Photoallergic: This is rare and is a result of the drug joining with a protein in our body. The body then tries to fight this combination off by creating an allergic reaction. Thiazide drugs and Bactrim are known to cause these problems.

Hats: People who golf, yacht, and fish, listen up. Too often, we forget the scalp. The ears and the nape of the neck need protection too. Hats should have at least 7.5 centimeters (approximately 4 inches) width at the brim to provide adequate protection. The best hats are those with a 360-degree brim, 4-inches-wide and with a neck flap. Believe it or not, hats are also rated with an SPF ranging from 0 to 7. The higher the rating, the better.

Sunglasses: It is important to know that the eyes are affected by the sun's rays too. Dark glasses do not guarantee protection. In fact, dark glasses, without appropriate treatment of the glass, can dilate your pupils and cause more UV rays to reach your retina. Orange/yellow lenses that offer the best reflection of the sun's rays are most recommended. Wrap-around types are the best.

UV Index

The UV index provides a method of forecasting the risk of overexposure to UV rays.

This is a complicated calculation, so it is fortunate for us that the math whizzes at the National Weather Service do this for most zip codes in the United States. Once they do the hard work the EPA (Environmental Protection Agency) publishes this information. This is a valuable tool for planning sun-safe outdoor activities.

You can get this information from the EPA website or download the free UV Index app to your Smartphone.

The UV Index ranges from:

0–2	Low danger for the average person from the sun's rays
3–5	Moderate risk of harm
6–7	High risk of harm
8–10	Very high risk
11+	Extreme danger

The Shadow Rule: An easy way to tell how much UV exposure you are getting is to look at your shadow. If your shadow is taller than you are (in the early morning and late afternoon), your UV exposure is likely to be lower. If your shadow is shorter than you are (around midday), you are being exposed to higher levels of UV radiation. Seek shade and protect your skin and eyes.

DIAGNOSIS
AND TREATMENT OF
MELANOMA

FOUR

THE DOCTOR'S VISIT

What do you do next if you find a new mole that's worrisome, or you're concerned about a suspicious mole that's changed recently?

You don't want to be an alarmist (stress isn't good for us), but it's important to have these moles evaluated. The only way to be sure that a mole is a melanoma is to have a pathologist look at it under a microscope. This requires a procedure called a biopsy. It's always better to be safe and get a biopsy. Even the best doctors find it difficult to diagnose melanoma just by looking at it. A trained professional can tell what is suspicious, and what is not through visual inspection. Only a biopsy can confirm a melanoma or its absence with absolute certainty. It's crucial that you see a doctor with specialized training in skin cancer and melanoma if you have, or suspect you might have melanoma.

THE DOCTOR'S EXAM—WHAT TO EXPECT

The first step your doctor will take is to collect information by reviewing your full medical history. The doctor will ask you when the mark first appeared, and whether it has changed in size or appearance. You might be asked the following questions:

- Has anyone in your family had skin cancer?
- Has anyone in your family had other cancers (such as breast, ovarian, pancreatic cancer, lymphomas or leukemia)? This may yield clues to your genetic predisposition to the disease.
- Have you been exposed to tanning beds?
- Have you been sunburned in your life?
- How much time do you spend in the sun?
- What medications are you taking?
- Do you have any other health issues?

During the physical exam, your doctor will note the size, shape, color, and texture of the area(s) in question and if you have experienced any bleeding or scaling. Your doctor will then check every inch of your body for spots and moles that could be related to skin cancer. The doctor may also feel your lymph nodes (small collection of immune system cells that are about the size of a pea), under the skin, in the groin, underarm, near the abdominal area, or close to the suspicious mole/growth. Enlarged lymph nodes might suggest that any melanoma might have spread. The other areas for examination are the abdomen, neck, mouth and eyes to be sure it hasn't spread.

If your exam is with a highly trained dermatologist, it may also include cutting edge techniques such as dermoscopy, also known as dermoscopy epi luminescence microscopy (ELM), or surface microscopy. These enable the doctor to examine the spots on the skin more clearly/carefully. The doctor uses a dermoscope, which is a special magnifying lens and light source held near the skin.

You may also have a digital or photographic image of the suspicious spot. These tests can improve the accuracy of finding skin cancers early. These tests can help distinguish benign lesions from cancerous ones sometimes without the need for a biopsy. This is when you need to listen to your instincts. If you feel strongly about a mole, have it biopsied. It's better to be safe than sorry, and just about every doctor will agree that most patients find these suspicious moles themselves, and self-skin checks combined with an astute doctor, is a winning team.

THE SKIN BIOPSY

Every diagnosis begins the same way, with a thorough skin exam under the bright lights in your doctor's office. If your doctor thinks he/she sees melanoma or anything that might look suspicious, their goal is to remove it either in part or completely during the biopsy. A biopsy is nothing more than removing a sample of skin from the suspected area, and examining it under a microscope.

Biopsies are considered a minor procedure and the risks are slight but it is a procedure, and you should keep a few things in mind. The most common risks are bleeding and infection. Bleeding is more of a problem if you have a clotting disorder. It's critical that you tell your doctor if you are taking blood thinners, aspirin or other medications that might have an effect on bleeding.

One crucial thing to consider before any procedure is that there are supplements that can affect bleeding, and you need to let your doctor know exactly what you're taking. See the following list of which supplements affect bleeding, and check with your doctor for a more detailed list.

> Omega-3 (all sources including Chia seeds)
> Flaxseed
> Glucosamine and Chondroitin
> Saw palmetto

Dong Quai
Feverfew
Vitamin E
Willow bark - Natural Aspirin
Garlic tablets
Ginger
Ginseng (All)
Echinacea
Goldenseal

WARNING: These supplements can be dangerous, and can cause serious complications or drug interactions during surgery. You'll find the complication listed next to supplement name.

Ginkgo Biloba: Seizure, heart attack, stroke
Ephedra–Ma Huang: Seizure, heart failure, stroke
St John's Wort: Heart failure
Kava: Coma
Valerian: Heart failure, delirium
Licorice: Bleeding in the brain and spinal cord

Discontinue these supplements at least 2 weeks before surgery, or as suggested by your physician.

By sharing all these facts with your doctor, they can deal with excess bleeding preventatively, or have you stop taking your medications or supplements for a few days before a biopsy. Don't underestimate the impact supplements and herbal remedies can have on bleeding. When in doubt, don't take them.

There are many different types of biopsies that can be used to biopsy skin. Some tumors may be too large, or may be located in a hard to reach area on the body or in a cosmetically important part like your face. The type of biopsy your doctor decides to use depends on the area the suspicious mole is located on your body, as well as the size of the growth. Different biopsies leave different size scars. Most biopsies leave small scars but are nothing to worry about when thinking about the big picture. If you're concerned about scarring, talk to your doctor before they do the biopsy.

Skin biopsies are done with local anesthesia, which numbs the area. The anesthesia is injected into the area with a very small needle. You'll feel a tiny quick needle prick, and possibly some stinging as the medicine is injected. You shouldn't feel pain during the biopsy.

Are there any other risks I should be aware of? Infection is uncommon. However, it's a good idea to tell your doctor if you are ill or not feeling well. Certain illnesses can increase the chance of infection and you may be asked to take antibiotics before the biopsy or procedure.

Another risk is an allergic reaction to the local anesthetic. The risk is extremely low, but you should let your doctor know about any allergies you might have before and after the procedure, so they can make note of it and better protect you.

Keep in mind that biopsies are used as a diagnostic tool and are not an adequate treatment for melanoma. It's critical that you return to your doctor after your biopsy to get your diagnosis, and they can guide you through the next steps that are needed for treatment.

TYPES OF BIOPSIES

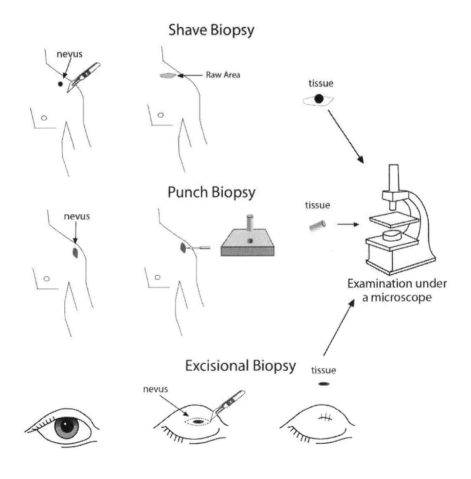

Shave Biopsy: A shave biopsy is another way to take a skin biopsy. The area is numbed the same way as with a typical biopsy. The doctor shaves off the top layers of skin (epidermis and most superficial part of the dermis), using a surgical blade. Shave biopsies are useful in diagnosing many types of skin diseases, and may be used to sample moles when melanoma risk is very low.

Punch Biopsy: The punch biopsy is used when a deeper sample of skin is needed. If the mole is small (3–4 millimeters diameter), and they only need a small piece to sample, the punch biopsy is the better choice because it removes a cylinder shaped piece of skin. Punch biopsies are done using a tool that looks like a round cookie cutter or large hole-punch. Once the skin is numb, the doctor manually rotates the punch biopsy tool on the surface of the skin until it cuts through all of the layers of the skin. Most punch biopsies only require a stitch, and sometimes only a piece of adhesive tape can be used to close the wound. The wound usually heals completely in a week or two. The punch removes enough skin for the pathologist to make a thorough examination of the mole/tissue, to make a judgment call.

Excisional Biopsy: Excisional biopsies are for skin lesions and moles that are larger than 4 millimeters, and it's necessary to take a broader skin sample to biopsy. An excisional biopsy is another surgical technique that's done using a local anesthesia and uses a scalpel in attempts to remove an entire lesion. Excisional biopsies can sometimes be performed by a skilled dermatologist in an office setting, or by a surgeon. If the mole is small enough, excisional biopsies require few stitches and heal in a week to 10 days. Most doctors use dissolving stitches that are excellent for healing, scar less, and save you time because you don't have to run to the doctor to have the stitches removed.

Most large moles are usually removed with either punch or excisional biopsies, and only a portion of the lesion is removed so that the suspicious looking area can be looked at. This allows the pathologist to examine the tissue thoroughly, make a diagnosis, and decide what the next step should be without being too aggressive with first removal.

Excisional biopsy is generally preferred if melanoma is suspected because it removes the entire tumor and a very small margin of normal tissue. It gives the pathologist the best chance to estimate the thickness of the melanoma, if it's present. However, this is not mandatory.

Fine Needle Aspiration Biopsy:

Fine Needle Aspiration

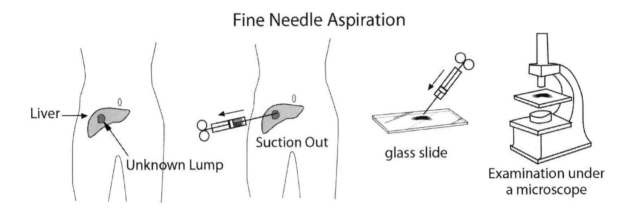

Liver → Unknown Lump   Suction Out   glass slide   Examination under a microscope

Fine needle aspiration biopsy, or (FNA), is not used on suspicious moles. FNA is a special biopsy technique that's sometimes used to diagnose melanoma in large lymph nodes that are close to the melanoma or lumps that may have melanoma cells in them. It can also be used for swellings inside the body, such as a lump in the liver so your doctor can look for metastasis.

This FNA procedure is done under local anesthetic and rarely causes discomfort, with minimal, if any, scarring. A large syringe is used with a thin, hollow needle to remove (suck out) very small tissue fragments. Sometimes it's necessary to insert the needle several times to obtain a tissue sample. Believe it or not, these needles are smaller than the needles used for blood tests. If the lymph node is near the skin, the doctor may be able to feel well enough to guide the needle into the questioned lymph node. If the lymph node is deeper, or cannot be felt, a computed tomography (CT) scan or ultrasound is used to guide the needle. The CT or ultrasound is also used for lumps deep inside the body. Once the tissue sample is collected, it's placed on a glass slide and examined under a microscope to be looked at by a trained pathologist called a cytopathologist or a cytologist, to examine. These experts can identify cancers by looking at a small number of cells versus looking at a large area of tissue.

IT'S PERFECTLY OKAY TO ASK FOR A 2ND OPINION!

BIOPSY FLOW CHART

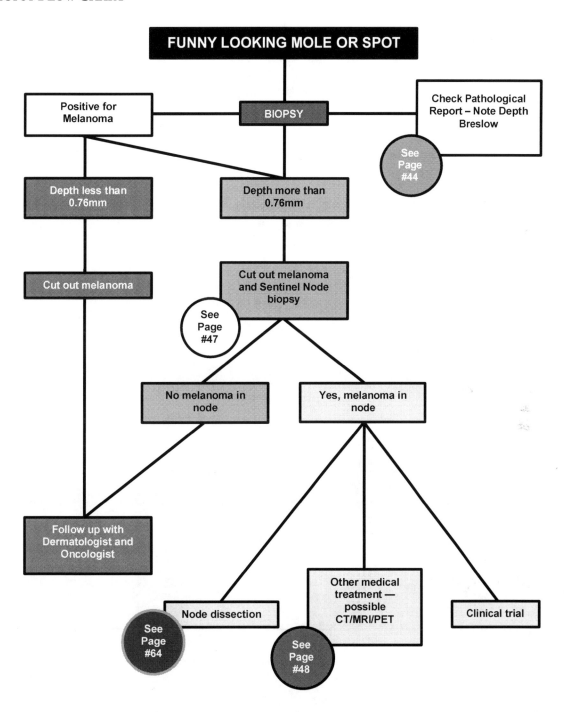

THE PATHOLOGY REPORT

DECIPHERING THE PATHOLOGY REPORT

If you are like most people once you've received a diagnosis of melanoma, the instinct is to run to the Internet and Google melanoma. This usually results in an avalanche of information that is sometimes overwhelming, even for medical professionals.

The best place to start your journey is your pathology report. This is the most significant document in your journey to fight melanoma.

I cannot emphasize the importance of this document enough because it gives you, in one fell swoop, a vast treasure trove of information about your melanoma, its behavior, the treatment, and prognosis. In short, a plan for the rest of your life. *It's that important.*

So let's see if we can break it down into bite-size pieces. Here is a model of how a pathology report looks:

Clark level
Breslow level
Vascular invasion
Mitotic rate

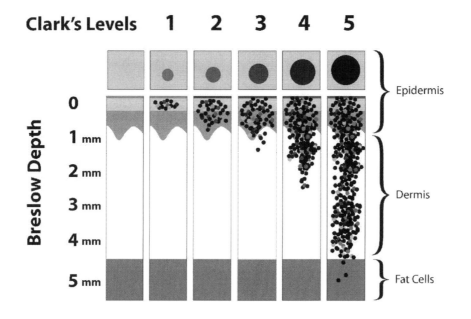

As you can see from the picture, an increase in the number of Clark or the Breslow, indicates the melanoma cells shown by dark dots has gone deeper into the tissue.

So what do the Clark and Breslow levels mean, and why are there two of them?

The Clark level was the first to be used to show how deep the melanoma was.

There are five Clark levels. You can follow along using the picture.

- Clark 1 is when the melanoma is confined to the skin
- Clark 2 is when the melanoma has gone to the dermis
- Clark 3 is when the melanoma is at the junction of the two halves of the dermis
- Clark 4 is when it is in the deeper part of the dermis
- Clark 5 is when it is in the fat

Clark level 4 is NOT the same as Stage 4 melanoma.

A problem arose when pathologists from around the world couldn't exactly tell the middle of the dermis from the lower half of the dermis. This was mainly because the skins of different people have different thicknesses. Even in the same person skin from various parts of the body have differences in the thickness of the dermis.

To ensure uniformity of diagnosis the Breslow level is widely used, which is a measure of the distance a melanoma has gone into the skin from a standard point of the surface. The distance is measured in millimeters or mm for short.

A millimeter is approximately 1/25th of an inch. With the use of a measurement like this, it becomes very easy to understand the depth to which the melanoma has gone regardless of where.

The reason both of these are still reported is because some doctors are used to the old system, and the Clark level helps to visualize the depth better than just a number in millimeters mentally. Thus, it is only a matter of convenience.

The Breslow number is the most important number in the pathology report and all the treatments that follow. It also gives you a very strong clue to your prognosis.

The mitotic rate is an indication whether the melanoma cells are dividing. It is usually expressed as a number per square millimeter. The higher the number, the faster the multiplication of the cells. A higher number, say, "12" versus "1" is not a good sign.

Vascular invasion indicates whether the melanoma cells have invaded the blood vessels. Sometimes the pathologist may suggest they see invasion of the lymphatics, which are thin cobweb-like channels that drain a filtrate of blood. Invasion of the blood vessels or the lymphatics is, generally speaking, not a good sign.

WHAT IS TNM STAGING?

The TNM staging was designed to let doctors the world over compare apples to apples. This produces a uniform description of a melanoma. The reason this is used is because the treatment, prognosis and characteristics of the tumor can be compared throughout the world, so there is no confusion about what is being described.

Here is a hypothetical example: Say a doctor in Australia describes a melanoma as advanced when it was 2 millimeters thick while a doctor in the United Stated calls a 10-millimeter melanoma as advanced. You can imagine the confusion. The Australian doctors could say their treatments worked for advanced melanoma while the doctor in the United States, going by his definition of advanced (which is actually five times worse) finds his advanced melanoma patients are not responding to the treatment at all and wonders why. Avoiding this kind of confusion is precisely the reason the TNM staging system was introduced.

The T stands for tumor, N stands for nodes (i.e., whether lymph nodes are involved or not), and M stands for metastasis. The T part in the case of melanomas refers to the thickness of the melanoma in millimeters or mm, for short.

The stage of a melanoma is determined by an assessment of T+N+M.

Thus, if you had a T1 melanoma that was 0.5 millimeters thick with no nodes (N0) and no spread (M0), you would be a stage 1.

Doctors use two forms of this staging system. A clinical TNM, which is done after a thorough clinical exam of the patient, and a pathological TNM which is done after surgery is completed and all the biopsy results are known. The pathological TNM carries more weight since it is more comprehensive and has more information.

Thickness of the melanoma and the extent of resection: Among the most commonly asked questions are:

- How do you know how much to take out?
- How deep do you go?
- How do you know you got it all?

The amount of tissue removed around a melanoma depends on the Breslow thickness. For a melanoma in situ, approximately 5–7 millimeters around the visible margins would be removed.

In this case, only the removal of tissue under the melanoma is limited to the level of the skin because the melanoma is restricted to the skin only and has not spread.

- 1 millimeter or less: Remove 1 centimeter (approximately ½ inch of tissue around the melanoma)
- 1–2 millimeters: Remove 1–2 centimeters (approximately ½–1 inch) depending on the body site
- 2–4 millimeters or more: Remove 2 centimeters (approximately an inch)

The depth of tissue removed is relatively standard. The surgeon removes all the tissue underneath the melanoma that is above the envelope of tissue called the deep fascia. The deep fascia is like a blanket that separates the muscles from the skin. Some surgeons may choose to remove part of this blanket to ensure that no melanoma cells are left behind.

As you can imagine, the actual thickness of the tissue can vary depending on the location of the body. For example, where there is no fat, such as the eyelids, the tissue removed is very thin. On the other hand, on the back or the abdomen, where there is more tissue, the specimen will be thicker.

If the surgeon uses these guidelines, for 95–99 percent of the cases, he can be sure that all of the tumor has been removed. These guidelines were established by studying thousands of cases and following them for many years, so we now know they are extremely reliable guidelines.

The need for sentinel node biopsy depends directly on the Breslow depth.

Now, do you see how important it is?

THE PATHOLOGY REPORT

> ➢ Tells the surgeon how much normal tissue to remove
> ➢ Tells the surgeon how deep to go when cutting the melanoma out
> ➢ Tells the surgeon whether a patient should have a sentinel node biopsy
> ➢ Tells the surgeon if the patient may need additional medication
> ➢ Tells the surgeon your prognosis (the chances of you dying in the next 5-10 years)

TESTS FOR MELANOMA

It's hard to believe in the 21st century there is no blood or X-ray test that is specific for melanoma. Unfortunately, it is true. There are no specific tests for melanoma. Doctors, however, may get some or all of these tests depending on the stage of the disease. The commonly used tests for melanoma are:

Imaging Tests: These are tests that take pictures (images) of your body or particular body part being studied such as an X-ray, CAT scan, MRI or a Lymphoscintigram for a sentinel node biopsy.

Blood Tests: The most commonly ordered test is the LDH (not LDL, which is related to cholesterol and has nothing to do with melanoma). This stands for Lactate DeHydrogenase, a blood test that is used to tell if there is evidence of spread elsewhere. Unfortunately, it is a very crude test and is indicated only in certain circumstances and certainly not as a routine test.

IMAGING TESTS

> Chest X-rays – routine
> Lymphoscintigram – not routine
> A CAT scan (Computer Assisted Tomography) – not routine
> An MRI (Magnetic Resonance Imaging) – not routine
> A PET scan (Positron Emission Tomography) – not routine

Why Do I Need Imaging Tests? Don't let these fancy terms make you nervous. Imaging tests are nothing more than pictures of the inside of your body. They are used mainly to look for metastasis to the lymph nodes and other organs. Each imaging test has its strong point or strength, which is why your doctor may choose one over another. Here is a short explanation to explain what each test does. Imaging tests are not always used for patients with early stage melanoma.

Chest X-rays are one of the most common and frequently used. Chest X-rays help determine whether melanoma has spread to the lungs.

Chest X-ray: A chest X-ray serves two purposes. It is a very crude test to see if the melanoma has spread to the lungs. Secondly, it will help provide the anesthesia doctors with valuable information if you are undergoing surgery and need sedation or general anesthesia.

Why Aren't Chest X-rays Used for All Melanomas? Because sometimes X-rays find perfectly harmless spots unrelated to the melanoma. Investigating these red herrings sometimes results in a wild goose chase and can cause more harm than good.

What Are CAT/CT Scans? Why Are They Better Than X-rays? CT (Computed Tomography Scan, or Computer Assisted Tomography) is just a sophisticated machine that takes multiple X-rays of your body. What makes it more complex is that the CT scan machines combine the X-rays to make a 3D picture. This picture can show, in very great detail, what's going on in the soft tissues and the internal organs. CT scans can also be helpful in determining whether the lymph nodes or organs are enlarged, which might be caused by the spread of melanoma. CT scans are better than standard X-rays when it comes to identifying whether or not melanoma has spread to the internal organs.

In the CT scanner, the machine takes many pictures as it rotates around you. A computer then combines these pictures into detailed images of the part of your body that's being studied. Standard X-rays take only one picture. CAT/CT scans are more thorough, so they take longer than regular X-rays.

Contrast solutions (special dyes) are sometimes used for CAT/CT scans and are administered either by having you drink a solution or through intravenous (IV) injection. The injection may cause an allergic reaction such as hives, itching, and minor swelling, which are rarely severe. It's important to let your doctor know if you have ever had a reaction to the contrast material used for X-rays. Some of the more severe reactions are trouble breathing and low blood pressure.

You'll be asked to lie still on a table during this test while the table moves in and out of the scanner, which is shaped like a donut that surrounds the table.

Another type of CT scan that's now available in many medical centers is called a Spiral CT or Helical CT. This type of CT uses a faster machine that operates/works the same way a standard

CT does, except it takes the pictures faster. This is more helpful than you think, as most of us can't sit still very long. It reduces the chance the images will be blurred because of our movement, or breathing motions. The Spiral CT also exposes patients to less radiation, and that's always a good thing.

What About an MRI? MRI is short for Magnetic Resonance Imaging. Magnetic Resonance Imaging, or MRI, is a painless and safe diagnostic procedure that uses radio waves and strong magnets, instead of X-rays, to take and give detailed images of soft tissues of the body. These radio waves are absorbed by the body, and released in a pattern formed by certain diseases or the type of body tissue. A computer then translates these patterns into detailed images of the part of your body being studied. Contrast materials (special dyes) are used less often with MRI's, but when used, they are usually injected. MRI's are especially good at looking at the brain and spinal cord.

The MRI is a long narrow tube that you lie very still in while pictures are being taken. Some find this uncomfortably confining and experience anxiety and fear (aka claustrophobia). It will help you to rehearse your distraction techniques or you might just relax and enjoy the quiet time. Fortunately, thanks to recent advancements in technology, there are newer, more open, MRI machines. If needed or preferred you can search for one in your area but it's more helpful to spend your time strengthening yourself mentally versus allowing fear to dominate you. The MRI does make loud buzzing, clanking noises, so if you're sensitive to loud noise, you may find it disturbing at times. Some places provide earplugs. I know a patient who sang her way through and it not only made her relax but she brought laughter to the people administering the test, and nothing is more healing than a good laugh.

The MRIs use very powerful magnets. It is vital that you tell the doctor or technician performing the MRI if you have any metal in your body. Metals such as joint replacements, metal plates and even things you may forget or are embarrassed about (nipple rings for instance).

Sometimes tattoos, which contain very, very small amounts of metal can be heated up by the magnetic field and can cause burns.

You will need to change into the clothes the MRI Center provides so that you are not harmed by unknown metal particles in your personal clothes.

What Are PET Scans? Positron Emission Tomography (PET scan) is a nuclear medicine, functional imaging technique that produces 3D images of the functional processes of the body.

For a PET scan, you receive an injection of glucose, which is a form of sugar that contains radioactive atoms. Cancer cells in the body absorb this radioactive sugar much more than normal cells. As a result, the areas that have cancer cells will glow brighter. A special camera then creates a picture of areas of the radioactivity in the body. PET scans, unfortunately, are not as detailed as MRI or CT scans but can provide helpful information about your whole body, particularly at the cellular level, which other tests cannot measure. In some centers, the PET scan is done along with a CAT scan (sometimes called a PET-CT) to get a better idea of exactly where the increased radioactivity (i.e., the cancer cells) are located. The CAT scan done along with a PET scan is usually not as detailed or sensitive as a regular CT scan.

PET scans are also used when your doctor thinks cancer may have spread but isn't sure exactly where. It's used most often for patients with advanced melanoma. The amount of radioactivity used is small. The downside is that areas of inflammation (say you had a boil on your skin) may also light up exactly as if it was a melanoma. Also, not all melanoma cells are active in absorbing this radioactive glucose.

OTHER TESTS

> **These tests are not very specific or sensitive so many authorities do not recommend their use in early stage melanomas.**

There may be tests that your doctor orders that may be only indirectly related to the melanoma such as:

CBC (Complete Blood Count): A complete analysis of the red blood cells, white blood cells, and cells called platelets that help in blood clotting, as well as the hemoglobin levels in your blood.

Serum electrolytes, Urea, and Creatinine: This is a measure of the various elements in your blood, and the capacity of your kidney to excrete anesthetic, or other drugs (urea and creatinine). These are used with certain people who undergo anesthesia, to ensure the safe administration of anesthetics.

Electrocardiogram: If you are older or have a history of heart disease, your doctor may order an electrocardiogram for the same reason.

Some of these tests may also be used by Medical Oncologists (the doctors who treat cancers, including melanomas by medicines as opposed to surgery), to manage their treatments.

SUMMARY: BEFORE SURGERY

➢ Doctor's visit: Biopsy of funny looking mole resulting in pathology report of melanoma

➢ If the surgeon did not do the original biopsy, you will be sent for a consultation with a surgeon

➢ The surgeon will talk to you about the actual surgery and determine if you need additional tests (blood or imaging)

➢ Once the tests are completed, the surgery is performed

FIVE

SURGERY FOR MELANOMA

The most common treatment for melanoma, if one went strictly by numbers is surgery. Going further along this line, the most common form of surgery for melanoma is an excision of the melanoma. This refers to cutting out the melanoma with a margin of normal tissue to ensure that all of it has been removed. The removal of this rim of normal tissue is to make sure that the melanoma does not come back in the same spot.

CUTTING OUT THE MELANOMA

Surgery is still the most important part of the treatment plan for a melanoma. When used appropriately, it can be curative for a vast majority of the melanomas. The keyword is 'appropriately'. Surgery is useful only for melanomas that are limited to a certain area or site. It cannot be used as a cure for melanoma that has spread to multiple sites or organs in the body. Sometimes a surgeon may remove a melanoma even though it has spread elsewhere, either to reduce pain or remove an area of infection. However, this is not a cure.

Four of the most commonly asked questions are:

1. How much healthy tissue around the melanoma should the surgeon remove?
2. How deep do you go?
3. How do you know you got it all?
4. How will the hole caused by the melanoma removal be filled?

How much healthy tissue around the melanoma should the surgeon remove?
The amount of tissue removed around a melanoma depends on the Breslow thickness.

For a melanoma in situ, approximately 5–7 millimeters around the visible margins.

In this case, only the removal of tissue under the melanoma is limited to the level of the dermis because the melanoma is confined to the skin only and has not spread.

- 1 millimeter or less: Remove 1 centimeter (approximately a ½ inch of tissue around the melanoma)

- 1–2 millimeters: 1–2 centimeters (approximately ½–1 inch) depending on the body site
- 2–4 millimeters or more: 2 centimeters (approximately an inch)

How deep do you go?
The depth that is removed is relatively standard. The surgeon removes all the tissue underneath the melanoma that is above the envelope of tissue called the deep fascia. The deep fascia is like a blanket that separates the muscles from the skin. Some surgeons may choose to remove part of this blanket to ensure that no melanoma cells are left behind. As you can imagine the actual thickness of the tissue can vary depending on the location of the body (for example if there is no fat as in the eyelids, the tissue removed is very thin). On the other hand, on the back or the abdomen where there is more tissue, the specimen will be thicker.

How do you know you got it all?
If the surgeon uses these guidelines, in 95–98 percent of the cases, he can be sure that all the tumor has been removed. The guidelines were established by studying thousands of cases and following them for many years so that we now know these are extremely reliable guidelines.

How will the hole caused by the melanoma removal be filled?
If the amount of tissue removed is small, then the cut can be closed directly.

If it is larger, your surgeon may choose to do a flap (if he or she is trained in Plastic Surgery). A flap is a technique where the neighboring tissue is moved in a special way to close the hole—a sort of surgical origami. The advantage of a flap is that tissue near the area of the cut is used, producing a good match. If your surgeon is not familiar with a flap, a plastic surgeon may be called to help. If you are lucky and you have a plastic surgeon who is also a surgical oncologist, you get two for the price of one.

In some cases, the hole might have to be filled by a piece of skin taken from another part of the body, say the thigh, and stitched around the sides of the hole to close it. This is called a skin graft.

In general, the cosmetic results of a flap are better than a skin graft. If you need a sentinel node biopsy to check if the melanoma has spread to your lymph nodes, you will have another cut where the surgeon takes out the lymph node. This can be in the neck, armpit or groin depending where your melanoma is located.

Remember: The excision and the lymph node biopsy (if required, a lymph node biopsy is performed) are done at the same time. Sedation or general anesthesia is required.

The surgeon sends the tissue that has been cut out to a pathologist to analyze the melanoma further. A pathologist is a doctor with special training who examines the specimen under the microscope to determine if it has been thoroughly removed, or whether there are other areas of melanoma in the tissue. They are also in charge of doing special tests on the lymph nodes if they have been removed, to determine whether melanoma cells have spread to them.

Most of the surgeries for melanomas are an outpatient procedure, which means you will be sent home the day of surgery. For some forms of surgery, you may be kept in the hospital, perhaps overnight, either to monitor other medical conditions or make sure your pain is adequately taken care of.

PREPARING FOR SURGERY

Remember, this is not an exam or test. Most, if not all of this, is good old plain common sense. If there is such a thing as a universal rule in this context, it is this, "If you don't know, ask."

The Location of the Hospital or Surgery: It might seem ridiculous to even list this, but I cannot tell you the number of times I have had patients land up at the wrong location or in the clinic thinking that was the same as the hospital. This is especially true if you live in a city that has many medical centers and outpatient facilities. Most hospitals or surgery centers call you the day before, to confirm the time and location of your surgery. If you haven't received a call, or if you are in doubt, call.

Make sure your surgeon's office and the hospital have at least two contact numbers where they can reach you. Also, ensure that the number listed is your most recent number.

Make sure you know where the parking area for the hospital is located and leave yourself time to park and get to the check-in.

Check the Date and Time of the Surgery: Patients are sometimes caught up with so many other concerns in their life that they may not remember the date and time of the surgery. Some-times the timing of the surgery might be changed if your surgeon has an emergency or the hospital decides to rearrange its schedule.

Medications: People are often confused about whether or not they should take their medications. Unfortunately, there is no blanket rule that covers all drugs. A few typical examples are given in this section.

Blood Thinners: Some drugs like Aspirin, Coumadin, or Plavix may need to be stopped a few days before surgery, as they prevent your blood from clotting. However, always check with your doctor about the advisability of stopping these drugs. For example, if you are taking Plavix because you had a heart stent put in recently, your surgeon may have to consult your cardiologist to come up with a specific plan to stop this drug, or not stop it at all. Similarly, if you are taking Coumadin to prevent a stroke, your surgeon may consult with your neurologist about switching you to a different type of blood thinner before the surgery, to minimize this risk.

Blood Pressure Pills: Generally, if you are on a regular blood pressure medication, your surgeon and anesthesiologist will want you to take it.

Insulin: Diabetics are a unique problem if general anesthesia is involved, especially if you are on insulin. This is because general anesthesia requires you to fast for 8 hours before the procedure.

Over the Counter Drugs: Most people forget to tell their surgeons about over the counter drugs like Motrin, garlic pills, or fish oil. All of these can thin your blood, and can cause problems during surgery.

Clothes: Keep the fancy clothes at home. Simple loose fitting comfortable clothes are best. Don't bring any valuables, cash or expensive equipment to the hospital.

Eating and Drinking before Surgery: Ask your doctor about the type of anesthesia you will have. If a procedure is done under local anesthesia, it is okay to have something light before the procedure.

Don't lie to your doctors if you accidentally took a bite of something or had a cup of coffee without thinking. This is dangerous if you are going to have sedation or anesthesia for the procedure. The reason it is dangerous is because with sedation, or general anesthesia, the stuff that you have eaten or drank can travel up your food pipe when you are lying down. They can then end up in your breathing tube, blocking your lungs so that you cannot breathe. Donuts or coffee (or even bagels or tea) are not meant to be in your lungs. What is worse is that they can inflame the lining of your lungs, and you could end up in the Intensive Care Unit for days. If the anesthesiologist tells you not to eat or drink before the surgery, follow this rule very carefully. In general, the anesthesiologists want your stomach empty for about 8 hours.

Mohs Surgery and Melanoma

People frequently ask me, "Why can't we do Mohs surgery for melanoma?". To answer this question, we must first explain what exactly Mohs surgery is. Mohs surgery, named for the surgeon Frederick Mohs, is a technique where the growth (cancer) is removed with a small margin of healthy tissue. This tissue is then examined by the operator, usually a dermatologist, under the microscope, by freezing the tissue and then cutting thin slices of the margin to look for cancer. If he finds one side (say, a part of the right side of the tissue removed) of the cut tissue has a bit of cancer, he cuts out more of the right side of the patient's skin area that may have more cancer. He then freezes it, slices it and looks under the microscope again to make sure all the cancer is removed.

This process is repeated until there is no more cancer seen under the microscope. Thus, the point of Mohs is that only the barest amount of tissue required to clear the cancer is removed.

This is particularly useful in certain types of skin cancers—squamous cell cancers or basal cell cancers. It is also useful in areas like the face where removal of a large amount of tissue may disfigure the patient. Thus, Mohs should be used only for specific cancers in specific areas.

Now, why not do that with melanomas?

The reason is that when the tissue is cut out and frozen, the normal melanocytes may change shape because of the freezing process and look exactly like melanoma cells. If this happens, the person cutting it out, freezing and examining the tissue may be fooled into cutting larger and larger amounts of tissue thinking that the melanoma is still present. The opposite may also happen when the operator might decide that the cells were normal and not take more tissue, thus leaving the melanoma behind.

This is why Mohs surgery is not used for melanomas.

Freezing does not affect the appearance of squamous and basal cells and therefore it is very easy to use Mohs for these skin cancers.

TIME REQUIRED FOR SURGERY

The surgeries are relatively short procedures. For example, if the surgery involves only cutting out the melanoma, most of these procedures can be completed in approximately an hour. The addition of a lymph node biopsy may add another hour, or an hour and a half to the procedure depending on the location of the lymph node, the size of the patient, etc. The more involved procedures such as the node dissections may take 2–3 hours.

ANESTHESIA FOR SURGERY

People who undergo surgery are most terrified by the prospect of pain during or after the surgery. You should know that in today's world anesthesia is an extremely comfortable and safe procedure.

The surgery itself can be done under different types of anesthesia. The various types of anesthesia techniques that can be used are described below. They are listed in order, starting with the easiest method to the more complicated ones.

- Local Anesthesia

  In this type of anesthesia, the surgeon injects a numbing medicine (like Novocain) into the area around the melanoma. Once he determines the area to be cut out is completely numb, the melanoma is removed, and the incision is closed. During this time, you will be wide-awake, and be able to talk with your doctor (if you want to), but you will not feel any pain. If you are one of those people who hates needles, are extremely nervous about them, or are sickened by the sight of blood or the smells of the operating room, then you are probably better off choosing another option.

- Sedation and Local Anesthesia

  Sedation involves the administration of a sedative medication intravenously while simultaneously numbing the area to be cut out. It is sometimes called twilight sleep. The anesthetist puts an IV in your arm and gives you a cocktail of medications that makes you drowsy and fall asleep, including painkillers, as well as drugs that help you forget the procedure itself. You may be aware of your surroundings, and hear snippets of sounds and conversation, but you will not feel any pain. Your surgeon will choose the type of anesthetic, depending on the type of your melanoma, and the need for additional procedures to be done at the same time (such as a sentinel node biopsy). Therefore just cutting out a melanoma may be done with a local anesthetic, but a sentinel node biopsy, or removing the lymph nodes from the armpit, will for most people require general anesthesia.

- General Anesthesia

  This is the most complete form of anesthesia available. In this type of anesthesia, you are completely unaware of your surroundings, and will not be able to experience any sensations. In short, you are knocked out. This method involves the placement of a breathing tube. You will not know or remember anything about the operation after you wake up. Once the procedure is completed, and you are awakened, you will be sent to the recovery room where trained nurses watch you for about an hour or so. They will monitor your vital signs, make sure you can eat, relieve yourself, talk and walk so that you can safely be sent home. After some types of melanoma surgery, you may be kept overnight in the hospital. Your surgeon may also decide to admit you to the hospital if they think you may need to be monitored because of problems such as heart disease or breathing problems.

- Nerve blocks or spinal anesthesia

  These are not commonly used methods for melanoma surgery. They are frequently used in other kinds of surgery such as orthopedic surgery (surgery of the bones).

In this method, the main nerves (in the case of the nerve block) to the arm, leg or the spine (in the case of a spinal anesthetic) are numbed with a numbing medicine (like Novocain). Once the anesthesia doctors are satisfied that you cannot feel any pain, they will let your surgeon proceed with surgery. They may also be able to give you sedative medication to make your time in the operating room more pleasant.

This procedure can be used only in special situations such as surgery of the arm, leg, or the lower part of the abdomen. The use of these techniques is variable in the United States and is highly dependent on the availability of anesthetists who are skilled in these methods. These may be helpful, for instance, in a patient who needs a general anesthetic or for some reason cannot have a breathing tube placed.

ANESTHESIA COMPARISON

	PROS	CONS
LOCAL ANESTHESIA	➤ Easiest ➤ Don't need someone to drive you home ➤ No need to starve the night before	➤ May require a few needle sticks before the area is numb ➤ Can hear, see and smell everything that's going on in the operating room
SEDATION	➤ More comfortable than local anesthesia alone ➤ You are not completely knocked out, so you recover faster than a general anesthetic	➤ You have to have someone drive you home ➤ You have to starve from the night before
GENERAL ANESTHESIA	➤ You are completely knocked out	➤ You have to have someone drive you home ➤ You have to starve from the night before ➤ Takes longer to recover

Nerve Blocks or Spinal

A nerve block, as the name suggests, is when the major nerve to the area is blocked by injecting a numbing medicine close to the nerve. Occasionally, the anesthesia doctors might leave a tube in the area to give more doses of numbing medicine.

A spinal anesthetic is a technique whereby a numbing medicine is injected into the area around the spinal cord. A similar technique called epidural anesthesia is used to help in the pain of childbirth. Both methods are rarely used for melanoma surgery, but it is good to be aware that they can be used if required.

SENTINEL NODE BIOPSY

This is a good place to discuss the topic of a sentinel node biopsy since it so heavily depends on the pathology report—namely the thickness of the melanoma.

The biggest problem with melanomas is that they can spread. The most common site to which they spread is lymph nodes.

Lymph nodes are little kidney shaped sponge-like tissues that filter fluid called lymph. In simple terms, lymph is like a diluted liquid part of the blood. It does not have red blood cells in it. Therefore, it has a clear or straw yellow appearance. It does have cells called white blood cells that help the body fight a variety of enemies such as bacteria, viruses, and even cancer cells. The lymph nodes have a large number of these cells, mostly a form of white blood cells, called lymphocytes that do the fighting.

Just as blood flows through arteries and veins, lymph flows through lymph vessels. These are extremely fine tubes that form a network under the skin that resembles a spider's web. They are usually so small that they cannot be seen with the naked eye.

So let's say you had a melanoma in your hand as shown in the picture on page 62. If the melanoma were to travel to the lymph nodes, it would most likely (greater than 99 percent of the time) go to the lymph nodes under the armpit. Similarly, if you had a melanoma on your knee and if it traveled, the first point it would stop would be the lymph nodes in your groin. You get the general idea.

Remember not all melanomas travel to lymph nodes—just a small percentage.

Now both you and the surgeon would very much like to know whether this spread has occurred. The easiest way of finding this out, though not accurate, is for the surgeons to feel for the lymph glands during the office visit. The reason this is not accurate is that a swelling in the lymph glands can be caused by things other than melanoma. An infection caused by a cut on your finger that you may have forgotten about is a good example.

The more accurate way of doing this, however, is to take out the lymph node and look at it under the microscope to see if there are any melanoma cells hiding out there.

Now, we have two problems

1. How does the surgeon decide which melanoma he is going to biopsy the lymph nodes?
2. How is he going to choose which lymph node to biopsy since there can be 30–40 of them under the armpit?

This is where the pathology report becomes so necessary.

The thickness of the melanoma, that is the Breslow number, is how that decision is made. If the thickness is more than 0.75 millimeters, I will do a sentinel node biopsy on the patient.

Other centers may use a different cut-off of 1 millimeter. To put it in different terms; if the thickness of the melanoma were 0.5 millimeters or 0.6 millimeters, most, if not all, centers in the United States or elsewhere, would not offer the patient a sentinel node biopsy.

The answer to the second question is—through a lymphoscintigram.

A lymphoscintigram (*limfo-sinti-gram*) is a particular test done by the radiologist to pinpoint the lymph node that the surgeon needs to take out.

See the diagram on the following page to see how it's done.

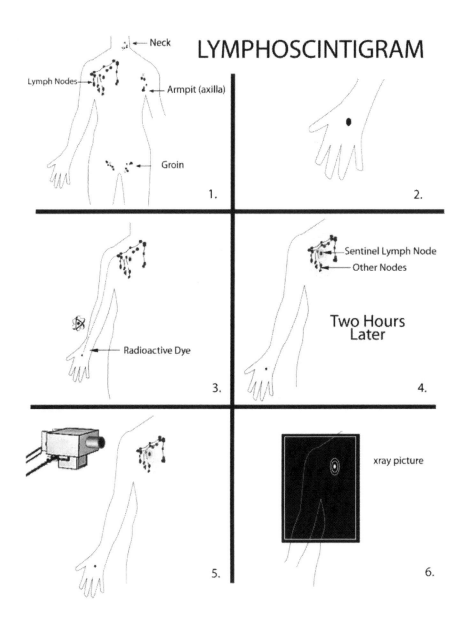

LYMPHOSCINTIGRAM

Frame #1: Distribution of major lymphatic sites.	Frame #2: Patient with melanoma of the hand.
Frame#3: To start the lymphoscintigram or dye test, radioactive material is injected around the melanoma which travels in the lymphatics (dotted line) to the lymph nodes.	Frame #4: The dye is concentrated in one (sometimes two) lymph nodes in 1–2 hours. This is the node the surgeon will biopsy at the time of operation.
Frames #5 & #6: An X-ray picture shows the position of the node because it is the only one that is radioactive. This is the sentinel node.	

Let's say you had a melanoma on your hand and the doctor decided to do a sentinel node biopsy. To do the biopsy, we need to figure out which node to cut out and send to the pathologist. For that, we do a lymphoscintigram. This test obviously has to be done before the surgery.

The first part is the injection of the radioactive dye. This may hurt a little bit.

The dye then travels through lymphatics (small channels that carry lymph, which is a filtrate of blood and are spread out under the skin like a meshwork) and reaches a particular lymph node. This is the sentinel node. For instance, if you had the melanoma on your arm, it might have gone to an entirely different node in the armpit. Sometimes it may go to two or very rarely three lymph nodes.

X-rays pictures are taken. This is the lymphoscintigram.

Sometimes it may take longer for the dye to get to the lymph node (perhaps as long as 2 hours)

You must remember that at the completion of this test, the surgeon will not be able to tell you whether the melanoma is in your lymph node or not. This can be done only after the lymph node is removed at surgery and looked at under the microscope. The lymphoscintigram is a road map for the surgeon, telling him which lymph node(s) to take out.

At the time of surgery, while you are asleep, the surgeon will inject the same radioactive dye into the site that is being cut out. He will locate the site of the sentinel lymph node using special cameras in the operating room and the road map of the lymphoscintigram. The node is now removed and sent to the pathologist. The melanoma is also cut out and reconstructed at the same time.

Do I really need to have a sentinel lymph node biopsy? What good does it really do? This is an excellent question, and I wish there were a simple answer.

The greatest advantage of doing a sentinel node biopsy is it gives the surgeon and the patient critical information about the prognosis. It also enables patients to be eligible for drug trials with new medicines that they might otherwise be excluded.

The rationale for the sentinel node biopsy is if we find one node that harbors a melanoma there may well be other lymph nodes with melanoma in the same area. In this case, the armpit that might have melanoma cells as well. Working on the principle that detecting the melanoma early is better for the patient, the surgeon might advise a second operation. Namely, a clean out of the lymph nodes in the armpit, a procedure called axillary node dissection. Along similar lines, if you had a melanoma in your face and there was a sentinel node in your neck that was positive for melanoma, the surgeon might perform a clean out of your neck lymph nodes on one side. This procedure is called a neck dissection. These are described later.

So what exactly is the concern? Despite the fact that it makes intuitive sense that taking out melanomas in lymph nodes early will save lives, this is not proven beyond doubt. Let's put it another way. If you had a sentinel node that was positive for melanoma, and you chose to wait and see if the other lymph nodes under your armpit grew from the melanoma, and then removed them, your life expectancy is exactly the same as if you had removed it earlier.

How does one make sense of this? The explanation that we currently have is if the melanoma cell had traveled to the lymph node, it means that the melanoma is a bad actor and it might have already have spread beyond the lymph nodes. So, taking out the lymph nodes early or late may not help in improving the survival.

I want to emphasize strongly that this is still a controversial topic because there may be a sub-group of patients that the logic of early removal of lymph nodes helps. It is to prove or refute this statement that many centers the world over are conducting trials to settle the matter once and for all. Unfortunately the results of the trials will not be known for a few years.

In the interim, most surgeons in the United States would offer the patient the lymph node dissection option rather than waiting. The reason being we cannot tell if you belong to the group that might be helped by removing all the lymph nodes once the sentinel node is found positive. If you have significant concerns about this, you should discuss this very carefully with your surgeon.

What are the disadvantages of a sentinel node biopsy? The disadvantages of the sentinel node biopsy are minimal. Bleeding, scarring, infection and pain at the site are common to all surgical procedures, and a sentinel node biopsy is no exception. Very rarely, there have been reports of lymphedema occurring even after the removal of a single or a few nodes. Once again, this is extremely rare, and I have not seen a problem in the many hundreds of cases I have personally performed.

What happens if the sentinel node is positive?

Lymph Node Dissections
The term lymph node dissection refers to the removal of all the lymph nodes in a certain area, such as one side of the groin, neck or armpit.

Neck dissection, axillary dissection or a groin dissection refers to the removal of lymph nodes in the neck, armpit or groin, respectively.

It is confusing because when you look at the term carefully there is no indication that the lymph nodes are removed—just dissected. It would perhaps be less confusing to call it axillary node removal and save everyone a lot of trouble and confusion, but that's life in the medical field.

So what happens if the sentinel node is positive? In the United States, most surgeons would advise you to undergo a node dissection of the area in which your sentinel node was found.

The logic of node dissection is that there is a chance the other lymph nodes in the same area (sometimes called basin) might also have melanoma cells in them. Once again, working on the principle that early removal of the cancer is beneficial, the surgeon advises removal of all suspicious nodes. However, there is a catch to this which we will address at the end of the chapter.

The other scenarios where a node dissection may be advised is if the doctor can actually feel an enlarged lymph node in one of these areas, and it is extremely likely that it is a metastatic melanoma, based on other tests and findings (even in the absence of doing a sentinel node biopsy). The third reason is when a melanoma appears in one of the lymph node areas mentioned previously, but no melanoma is detectable anywhere in the body. In other words, a primary site is never identified. This is called metastatic melanoma with an unknown primary.

How does this last scenario happen?

A melanoma appeared on the skin at some point in the past, but the body was able to fight it off at the site where it originally appeared. Some of the melanoma cells escaped, hid out in the lymph nodes, and for some unknown reason, started to grow. The word primary refers to the site where the parent melanoma is located. Surprisingly, the prognosis in these cases may be just as good, if not better because the body seems to have figured out a way of fighting off at least some of these cells.

General features of all lymph node dissections
A node dissection is a bigger deal than a node biopsy. It takes longer, is done under general anesthesia and is a more involved undertaking, both for the patient and the surgeon. The effects of a node dissection can and does have some long term consequences. These procedures may require an overnight stay in the hospital. They may involve the use of drains (clear plastic tubes that are temporarily placed under the skin to drain the extra fluid produced by the body). The following figure shows what a common drain called a Jackson-Pratt (JP for short) looks like.

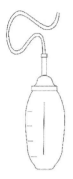

These procedures may require you to take a longer time off from work.

The fundamental principles of a node dissection are the same, regardless of the area. An incision (cut) is made over the area to be dissected. The skin is peeled back and the lymph nodes and fat are removed leaving behind vital structures like blood vessels or nerves. The skin is then stitched back, usually leaving a drain or drains that will be removed in a week or 10 days, rarely longer. As an example, removing the lymph nodes in the armpit, the axilla, is shown in these figures.

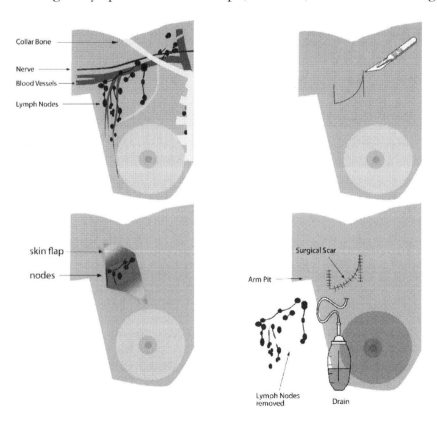

The technical term for this is axillary node dissection.

Note that the vital structures such as the blood vessels and nerves are preserved.

Bleeding, scarring (bad looking scars), infection, persistent numbness or pain, are common to all these procedures. Because the lymphatic channels are being disrupted, fluid might fill up the space where the lymph nodes were removed. This is called a seroma and may well be the most common complication of these procedures. It is precisely to prevent this that the drains are placed at the site, but seromas may form after the drains have been removed. Depending on the size of seromas, the doctor may choose to wait till the body absorbs the fluid or put in a needle and remove the fluid.

Certain side effects are unique to the area being dissected.

> **Neck dissection**
>> Stiffness of the neck
>> Numbness in the ear—men may cut themselves shaving and not know it

> **Groin Dissection**
>> The groin incisions can be made in different patterns as shown below

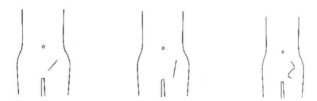

Lymphedema may be more commonly seen as a result of these procedures. It does not cause impotence or infertility. This appears to be a common question in men.

Axillary Node Dissection: There can be numbness on the inner side of the arm. This is common and is usually a result of the nerve to that part of the skin being cut. The surgeon sometimes has to cut the nerve on purpose, so as not to leave any cancer behind. This does not interfere with any function of the arm. Occasionally, this may hurt for a longer period of time and other types of medication may be prescribed to control the symptoms.

Lymphedema: This is a problem most patients and doctors fear most about node dissections.

Lymphedema is a condition whereby the lymphatic fluid, instead of traveling back into the blood supply, tends to hang around in the tissues and over time enlarges the limb. In other words, the leg becomes swollen. The exact cause is unknown. It is most common in the leg but can be seen in the arm as well. It is more frequently seen in obese females and may be made worse by radiation, massage therapy or pressure stockings. JOBST stockings are of significant help in keeping this under check. Recently surgeons have transplanted lymph nodes from other parts of the body into the affected limb to improve the situation. The benefits are just being studied.

Other than an increase in the size of the limb, there is an increased likelihood of infection in the limbs with lymphedema. This is usually caused by a form of strep infection.

Practical Tips to Prevent Lymphedema

- Gloves while washing dishes
- Control diabetes
- Gardening gloves
- Use opposite arm for blood draws
- Strep infection in hand (see doctor)
- Red streaks running up the arm (see doctor)
- Treat any infection in the affected limb aggressively
- Pressure Stocking
- JOBST stocking
- Keep limb elevated
- May present late (years) so don't slack off on the precautions

So what is the catch? The catch is that if you looked at 100 people undergoing node dissections for a positive sentinel node, only 20 percent of them would have more nodes that have melanoma cells in them. In other words, of the 100 patients, 80 of them will have had the dissection for no reason. Unfortunately, we have no way of predicting with any degree of certainty who will fall in the 80 percent group and who will fall in the 20 percent. There are many groups around the world studying this problem, but it will be a few years before we know the results.

AFTER SURGERY

COMMONLY ASKED QUESTIONS

Will I have stitches or staples?
Most doctors use stitches.

Will the stitches dissolve on their own?

The stitches under your skin will dissolve on their own. Most often, the ones on the skin that are visible will have to be removed.

Can I shower? Can I get the incision wet?

This depends on your surgeon's preference and practice. Some surgeons like to keep the incision dry until the stitches are removed. Other surgeons let you shower in a couple of days after the procedure and let the incision get wet.

How much pain will I be in?

This is a difficult question to answer as the threshold of pain is vastly different for each person. For the small excisions, the pain is usually minimal, including excisions with or without flaps or skin grafts. When the anesthesia wears off you may be helped by taking the pain medications prescribed. Some patients seem to do very well with Tylenol alone while others may need stronger pain pills like Percocet.

In general, a mild, moderate painkiller like Tylenol with codeine will suffice for the vast majority of the patients. The pain may be replaced by a dull ache in a few days which may or may not require any pain medication. Any pain that to your mind seems excessive, intolerable, or suddenly appears out of the blue may require a call to your doctor to check things and rule out any complications.

When can I resume my regular pills?

Usually the same or next day. If you are on blood thinners or Aspirin-like drugs, your surgeon may ask you to wait for a few days. It is best to check the timing of this with your surgeon.

How much time should I take off from work?

It depends on the type of work you do.

If, for instance, you had a melanoma removed from your arm and you lift heavy weights at work, it may be wise to wait a couple of weeks. This will decrease the amount of pain and swelling that might be caused by overexertion of the arm. Waiting will also prevent the stitches from breaking open, causing the healing process to be prolonged. On the other hand, if your job is that of a receptionist and did not involve lifting heavy weights, you could conceivably be back to regular work in a couple of days. As always, it is best to check the timing of this with your surgeon.

Will I need antibiotics?

For a vast majority of the cases of melanoma surgery, there is no need to take antibiotics after the surgery. The surgeon may choose to give you an antibiotic intravenously if the surgery is of the most extensive kind. If you have an artificial heart valve or hip, it may be wise to take antibiotics (by mouth) before the surgery, even if it is under local anesthesia.

How will I know if I have an infection?

The usual signs of infection are redness, fevers, chills, a sudden worsening of pain, and/or excessive warmth or drainage from the wound site.

When should I come back to see the doctor?

Usually, the surgeon will see you back within a week to 10 days, to examine the incision, make sure there is no infection, remove stitches and possibly discuss the results of the pathology report.

Will insurance cover my surgery?

Different insurance companies have different policies for co-pays and premiums. Generally, insurance will cover the cost of treatment. You should always call your insurance company to determine exactly how much you will be required to pay (co-pay) as a part of the operation, postoperative visits and subsequent follow-up and tests if required.

I love my exercise. When can I run, jog, or swim?

In general it's good to wait 2–4 weeks before doing anything strenuous, especially when the surgery is in an area that is subjected to physical stress as in the lower legs, arms or abdomen. Always check with your surgeon before you do this since there may be other factors that prolong the healing process such as diabetes, smoking or steroids.

Before swimming in the ocean, pool or lake make sure your surgeon gives you the go-ahead since bacteria can settle on partially healed wounds and cause an infection.

SCARS FROM SURGERY: HOW DO I GET THE BEST LOOKING SCAR?

People don't often realize that it takes nearly one full year for the scar to mature.

If you are lucky, the scars may begin to fade or become invisible within 6 weeks. More often, the scars usually tend to become thicker and redder, because of increased blood flow and new tissue deposition, for the first 6–8 weeks and then slowly start to fade away. Naturally, you cannot put your life on hold for that length of time. From a common sense point of view, it may be best to limit strenuous activity (gym running, etc.) for at least 2 weeks, sometimes as long as 4 weeks depending on the location and then slowly resume normal activities. Too rapid a resumption of strenuous activity may cause a persistent swelling in the area which may widen the scar. Or worse, the stitches might split and leave you with a gaping wound which certainly will not produce the scar of your dreams. Infections of wounds, in general, produce worse scars than non-infected wounds so you must be careful about swimming in the ocean or pool too soon.

Keep the scar protected from direct sunlight for 4–6 weeks. For some reason, this seems to darken the scar more.

One of the most commonly recommended methods to diminish or flatten a scar is the use of silicone sheets for times ranging from 8 to 12 or 16 weeks. It is not clear why they work. They can be applied directly to a healed scar, usually after the stitches are removed. They look like clear plastic strips or sheets and are available over the counter at most pharmacy stores. Any brand will work as well as the other. A variety of other creams and potions including shea butter and vitamin E have been touted as improving scars and people swear by them. Unfortunately, there is no proof that any of these work, and in some cases, may make matters worse.

This is as good of time and place as any other to talk about sensation in scars.

In the early weeks, it is common to get itching in the scars. This may be related to chemicals released by the white cells that are involved in the healing process. For several weeks or months after, feeling funny sensations is common in the scar. Sometimes it's a dull ache from excessive exercise, or sharp electric shock pains which last for only a few seconds. This is more than likely caused by regenerating nerves.

The key point here is that all these sensations are normal if they are present for limited periods. Anything that seems to persist for weeks or months will require medical attention.

It is also common to feel abnormal sensations in the scar during changes in the weather, as well as changes in color. For patients who live in the colder areas, this effect may be pronounced in the first winter or summer after the surgery.

Numbness in scars can occasionally be permanent. More often than not a patchy return of sensation is seen.

Keloid and hypertrophic scar: Occasionally, despite everything being done right, the scar might not look good. By that I mean, it may widen or thicken, or occasionally do both at the same time.

There are many reasons for this. The first thing to remember is that everybody heals differently. You may have an entirely different reaction to the stitches that are placed under the skin compared to your friend or family member. Also, remember that in cases where the melanoma is cut out, a piece of skin is removed. When the edges are pulled together the natural elasticity of the skin tends to pull the cut edges outward thus widening the scar.

This is not true for all types of surgery. For instance, in a C-section or an appendix removal, no skin is removed. So the edges fall back to where they were before the operation and there is no pull on the edges. Thus, these scars may look better.

The location of the incision and skin color also matter. Incisions involving removal of skin on the back generally produce thicker scars. Incisions near joints may widen, because of movement, compared to incisions on the forehead. People of color (Hispanic, African American, Indian or Oriental) tend to have more prominent scars, which may be due to increased pigment in the skin.

People sometimes erroneously call these scars keloids and they are wrong.

The scars which are limited to the region of the cut of the original scar and are a little more prominent are called hypertrophic scars. I suspect the reason people call them keloids is because it is easier to say than hypertrophic, which is a mouthful.

Keloids are rare cauliflower-like thickenings that spread outside the borders of the original scar. The reason some people get them is unknown. Once again, they are most common in people of color and will require particular forms of treatment.

SPECIAL SURGICAL PROCEDURES

SURGERY FOR METASTASIS
Occasionally, there may be situations where surgery is required for metastasis.

Such surgery is performed if there is a single or limited number of metastasis that can easily be removed without endangering the function of the organ. Some examples are single metastasis to the lung, liver, bowel, spleen or very rarely, the brain. Local recurrences may also be treated surgically. The thought is that compared to the medications which have unpredictable side-effects, surgery may be able to get rid of the tumor in a predictable fashion. Another example of this kind of surgery is when a metastasis, being treated with medication, grows despite increases in dosage or addition of other drugs.

Isolated limb perfusion and isolated limb infusion are reserved for those very rare situations.

- When the metastasis are limited to the limbs (either upper or lower)
- There is no evidence of metastasis elsewhere
- There are too many metastases in the limb to be cut out
- The metastases keep coming back in the limb without any evidence of spread elsewhere

How does it work?

The fundamental principle is to give very high doses of the medication only to the affected limb so that it is not toxic to the rest of the body. Let's take, for example, a patient with multiple melanoma metastases in the leg. The surgeon makes a cut in the groin and fishes out the two major blood vessels; the femoral artery that brings fresh blood to the leg and the femoral vein that takes the used blood back to the heart. A tube is placed in the artery and another into the vein. Very high doses of the chemotherapy drug are sent into the artery and the blood returning from the leg is removed through the vein without releasing it to the rest of the body. A tourniquet is tied around the upper part of the leg to prevent leaks. It is then recirculated for approximately 2 hours. In the isolated limb perfusion method, a pump is used to direct the flow.

The infusion process is much less invasive, involves placing the catheters in the vessels without major surgery and not using the pump at all.

As you can imagine these are very unique scenarios, and only a limited number of hospitals even offer this method of treatment.

QUESTIONS TO ASK
You may be so full of fear that you can't think straight, so bring a friend to your appointment for moral support, and make a copy of questions to bring with you. If you feel unsure about anything, you should ask about getting a second opinion.

FOLLOW-UP CARE

What next? What do you need to do to stay healthy after treatment for melanoma?

You'll be relieved when treatment is completed. This is the best time to focus on your health and wellness. It's going to take some time for your confidence to return, and once the recovery begins you'll start to feel normal again. It's not easy to stop worrying about whether cancer will return. This fear is very standard among survivors/thrivers. You can only place your focus in one area—choose healthful living.

Once your treatment is finished, no matter what stage melanoma you had, you will require ongoing care, which differs with every stage. Although there is no guarantee your melanoma won't come back, people learn to live with the uncertainty, and they get used to this new normal.

> *"Worry looks around, fear looks back, faith looks up, guilt looks down, but I look forward." - Unknown*

FOLLOWING THROUGH FOR A HEALTHIER YOU

After treatment is over, it's imperative to keep all follow-up appointments. The follow-up care is the best way to protect yourself. Your team will be checking for cancer recurrence and metastasis, as well as any possible side effects you may be experiencing. Don't be afraid to ask your health care team questions and to discuss your fears and concerns.

The follow-up care is on two different fronts. The reason for two separate sets of doctors following you is because they are experts in various fields. The skin doctor will make sure there are no new melanomas growing on your skin whereas the medical oncologist and surgeon will make sure the melanoma you had has not spread elsewhere.

Skin Doctor: This follow-up is for life. If you've had a melanoma, the skin doctor may have you come back as frequently as four times yearly. If you have lots of moles or atypical moles, your skin doctor may suggest you be seen more often.

The Medical Oncologist and the surgeon: How often you will need follow-up care depends on the stage of melanoma. Your follow-up care may include physical exams (don't forget your weekly skin exams) and lymph node examinations. Also, you may receive blood and imaging tests though these are limited.

Most typical follow-up schedules for thin or stage I or II melanomas, usually call for a 6-month physical exam for approximately 5 years after the surgery. Thicker melanomas might include physical exams every 3–6 months for 2–3 years, reducing to 6 months for the next 3 years. Most times after that, exams are done at least once a year.

Depending on your case, your doctor may also suggest chest X-rays to be sure your lungs are clear, and melanoma hasn't metastasized. He may also perform blood tests like the LDH to detect metastases, every 6–12 months. If you've had a more advanced stage melanoma, you may also receive other tests such as CT scans.

Depending on your location and the preference of your physicians, this may all be done by the Medical Oncologist or the surgeon or sometimes in tandem, alternating with the Medical Oncologist and the surgeon.

It's important you protect yourself by doing your regular weekly skin check. If you find a new lump or mole, it's important to see your doctor right away. You should also report symptoms that don't go away, such as pain, fatigue, cough, and loss of appetite. Melanoma can come back even 10 years later so follow-up will help to keep you safe.

Stage IV melanomas that have been removed or disappeared after treatment may have the same monitoring schedule as people who have had thicker melanomas. Most Medical Oncologists prefer to have these patients seen every 3 months for 5 years. For melanoma cases that are more difficult, your doctor will suggest a follow-up, based on your situation.

If you have had one melanoma, you may still be at risk for another melanoma, and need to be vigilant. It's also possible to develop other skin cancers. We cannot stress enough, consistent self-skin checks every week to be on the safe side. Also, avoid too much sun.

REMEMBER: There is nothing magical about the 5 year mark. In some cases, you may need to be followed up for longer periods.

SPECIAL SITUATIONS

Pregnancy: There is no evidence available at the time of writing that pregnancy worsens the prognosis of melanomas. If melanoma is diagnosed during pregnancy and it is too early to have the child, the removal of the melanoma can be performed under local anesthesia or sedation. Some patients would prefer to wait to do the sentinel node biopsy (if required) after the delivery.

Blood donation: Initial guidelines permanently barred people with melanoma from donating blood. The standards have now been relaxed in that the ban is not permanent. The exact answer depends on the stage of your melanoma and recurrence if any. It is best to check with the blood bank specifically regarding donation guidelines.

Transplantation and organ donation: The consensus is that patients who have previously been treated for melanoma should not donate organs. In 2005, the Canadian Society for Transplantation suggested that such a patient should wait 5 years before receiving a transplant and 2 years for a melanoma in situ. Once again, it is best to check with your transplant team regarding the most recent guidelines and whether you can be listed as a potential recipient.

STARTING OVER WITH A NEW DOCTOR

You may find yourself in a new doctor's office at some point. Doctor's move, retire, or you may move away. Whatever the reason, it's important to provide your new doctor with exact details of your diagnosis and treatments that you've received.

Be sure to provide the following information:

- Copies of pathology reports from any and all biopsies, as well as surgeries
- Copies of your operative report, if you had surgery
- If you were hospitalized, a copy of the discharge summary the doctor must prepare when you're sent home
- If you had radiation therapy, a summary of the type and dose of radiation that was administered, as well as where it was given
- If you had chemotherapy, or immunotherapy: a complete list of the drugs, dosages, as well as when they were taken
- Make personal notes on side effects you experienced, as well as your questions

Even though your cancer seems like a thing of the past, you should keep your medical insurance active. No one wants to think melanoma will return, but it is a possibility. The last thing you need to worry about is paying for your treatment.

SIX

MEDICATIONS FOR MELANOMA

No one likes the thought of being cut open. In a perfect world, there would be a pill for everything; weight loss, happiness—melanomas. An ideal world is a far cry from what we live in and that most certainly applies to melanomas.

I say *applies* because what was true even 5 years ago has changed in a most dramatic fashion for melanomas. While we are still a ways from perfection, we have at least found the path that will lead to it.

Rather than getting to the exciting part right away, I'm going to take you on a tour (virtual) showing you what *was available*, ending up with what *is available* now. Part of the reason for doing this is to give you an understanding of how slowly changes can come to a medical field. Despite the presence of new drugs, there still may be a role for the older ones, under the appropriate circumstances.

CHEMOTHERAPY – INTRODUCTION

When most people hear the word chemotherapy, their minds are filled with visions of people poisoned by drugs, losing their hair and appetite, and looking like a skeleton of their former selves. While some of these drugs may be used in melanoma treatment, the newer drugs are different in that they work, not by poisoning the cancer cells (and the patient's healthy cells), but by using the body's own system to fight the invaders.

Drugs like Interferon and Interleukin-2, which you will read about in the next few pages, are chemicals produced by your own body's immune cells to fight melanoma. Thus, although they are technically a form of cancer-fighting medicine, they are not the poisons of yesteryear. Therefore, they do not cause hair loss or an increased chance of infections.

The most recent drugs; such as Vemurafanib (trade name Zelboraf), Dabrafenib (trade name Tafinlar), Ipilumimab (trade name Yervoy), Pembrolizumab (trade name Keytruda), and Nivolumab (trade name Opdivo) are even more different than Interferon and Interleukin 2 (IL-2).

Vemurafenib, for instance, is a drug that can only be used in melanomas that have a mutation in a gene called B-raf. This is an example of a molecularly targeted treatment. Because it is so specific for the mutation, it does not kill any cells (normal or melanoma cells) that do not have this change.

Drugs like Ipilumimab (Ipi for short) and Pembroluzimab (Pembro for short) are radically different drugs in that they don't directly kill the cancer cells. Instead, they rev up the body's immune system and make the body fight cancer. In other words, they teach the body to fight cancer on its own. I have used the word cancer instead of melanoma because these drugs have shown promise in the treatment of other cancers; such as kidney cancer.

Let's start at the beginning.

CHEMOTHERAPY

For the last 35 years or so there were very few drug options for the treatment of melanoma. Chief among them was a drug called Dacarbazine, which to this day, remains the only chemotherapy drug (not biologicals or the newer drugs) approved by the FDA, for the treatment of melanoma. The drug can be given intravenously only and had to be repeated every 3–4 weeks. It is, in general, a well-tolerated drug but only 10–15 percent of patients respond to it and even if they do so, it is only for a limited period.

A significant advance in this area came with the development of an oral (pill form) form of Dacarbazine called Temozolomide (Temodar, Temodal—trade names). It worked just as well as Dacarbazine given intravenously and had the additional benefit of being able to penetrate the brain so that it could be used for brain metastases. It is important to realize that this drug did not prolong survival to a level exceeding Dacarbazine.

To improve options for patients with melanoma doctors, researchers tried a variety of other traditional chemotherapy drugs. A few of them are Vinblastine Paclitaxel, Lomustine, and Carmustine. Unfortunately, the results were no better than Dacarbazine and, in fact, some were worse.

THE BODY'S DRUG CABINET (ALSO KNOWN AS THE BIOLOGICALS)

After a prolonged drought, around the mid-1990's, two new drugs came to the market that in some ways pointed researchers once again to the prospects of using the immune system to fight melanoma.

Interferon Alpha: The first drug, Interferon, is a chemical produced by your body; namely the white cells. It was first discovered when scientists found that a human cell infected by a virus secreted a chemical that interfered with a second virus re-infecting the cell; hence the name.

The major difference between this medication (and Interleukin that we will discuss next) is that the medications do not kill the melanoma cell directly like Temozolomide or Temodar or any of the drugs in the previous section. Instead, these drugs stimulate the body's defense mechanisms to fight the invading cancer cells.

Interferon is now given, generally speaking, in a high dose phase which lasts about a month. This is followed by an 11-month period where the drug is administered by the patient to himself or herself, by an injection under the skin, usually three times weekly. This is very similar to the way diabetics administer insulin to themselves.

While it was initially thought to be a game changer, it is now known that the benefits of Interferon are marginal at best. There may be a tiny group of patients who may benefit from this treatment. The drug is not given to all patients with melanoma.

It is mainly directed to patients who have a very high risk of recurrence such as a broad or aggressive melanoma, or in the case of patients who have involvement of the lymph nodes only, without evidence of the melanoma having spread elsewhere. The logic behind the use of Interferon in this setting (sometimes called adjuvant therapy) is that there may be melanoma cells that may have spread elsewhere in the body that we just cannot see by any method we have. This, once again, is most likely to happen in the high-risk melanomas. By giving Interferon, we can use the body's defenses to flush out and kill these hidden melanoma cells so that they will not grow and pose a danger in the future.

There are significant side effects associated with the 11-month course of Interferon. The most common complaint that patients have is that it feels like they have the flu.

In a sense, this is very accurate since some of the symptoms we experience with the flu, like weakness or malaise (tiredness), is directly caused by the body secreting Interferon to fight the flu virus. A part of the reason for these symptoms is that the dose of Interferon given is several hundred times higher than what the body generates.

Unfortunately, however, unlike the real flu, these flu symptoms do not go away in a week. Some patients have found that drinking plenty of fluids or on occasion taking Tylenol before the injection may help relieve the symptoms. Other problems may include depression, a drop in white cells, nausea, diarrhea, and a low blood count resulting in tiredness from a lack of hemoglobin, among others. This list is by no means a comprehensive one, and you must check with your physicians if you have any concern.

Interleukin-2 or IL-2: Interleukin 2 is another chemical that is produced by the white cells in the blood. It acts by increasing the number of other white cells and the secretion of chemicals that help kill or neutralize melanoma cells. Unlike Interferon, IL-2 is given only as an intravenous injection. Interleukin-2 is given only for metastatic melanoma; that is melanoma that has spread elsewhere in the body. This is different from Interferon, which is given as a preventive measure rather than as a treatment.

This is a more toxic drug than Interferon and has to be administered intravenously. Most people have flu-like symptoms such as fever, chills, and joint and muscle aches and weight gain. A rapid heart rate, decrease in urine output, and a drop in blood pressure are also common. Also, you may have nausea, vomiting, and diarrhea. This may result in observation or resuscitation in the ICU (intensive care unit). IL-2 is a very unpleasant drug but with a good side.

The good thing about IL-2 is that it cures a small proportion of patients with metastatic melanoma, and the duration of the response can last for years.

BIO-CHEMOTHERAPY

Because of the less than encouraging results of these drugs when used alone, doctors decided to combine them to give melanomas a one-two punch. Thus, bio-chemotherapy was born, which is the combination of biological drugs (the bio part) and chemotherapy drugs that we just discussed. Despite some good initial results, the original promise was not borne out in later studies.

NEW DRUGS OF THE MELANOMA TREATMENT REVOLUTION

In this section, I am going to discuss three types of drugs, each of which acts by a different mechanism. The surprising thing about these medications is that they have been available only for the last 3 years or so (in some cases for a year). They have revolutionized the treatment of melanomas that have spread (i.e., the ones that cannot be surgically treated) and in some cases have been used instead of surgery. For those of us who have been in the field long enough this is nothing short of a miracle.

I am going to digress here and tell you a story about my *Come to Jesus* moment.

As I mentioned earlier in the book, I am very fortunate to be working at one of the world's premier medical centers, the Yale-New Haven Hospital. As a result, my patients have access to experimental drugs, years before the general population does, should these drugs prove effective and come to the market. Of course the experimental drugs might not work at all, but in the case of melanoma, something was always better than nothing.

One of my patients, let's call him Mr. B, came to my clinic a few years ago saying that his neck hurt.

Mr. B was a poster child for the 1960s; tie-dye t-shirts, antiwar tattoos, the works (we are Happies, not Hippies, as he liked to say). I had removed a melanoma from his scalp years ago and had not seen him after since he skipped his follow-up appointments. What I saw shocked me. He had large tumors in his neck the size of grapefruits, as well as others on his cheek and one over his jaw. I spoke to him about the urgency of the situation and the importance of immediate surgery.

He said, "Doc if I am going to die anyway, I might as well fulfill my dream of seeing Cuba before I pass on. Is there anything other than surgery you can offer?"

I would be lying if I said I took this calmly. I begged, pleaded, cajoled and threatened him, while trying to talk him out of his trip to Cuba, which to my ears sounded completely asinine given the gravity of the situation. Mr. B, however, was adamant. I therefore reluctantly signed him up for a trial with Ipilumimab (which was then experimental and had not yet reached the market), with the promise that he would return straight to my clinic after this Cuba business was completed. There goes another patient, I thought to myself, traumatized by this incident because we had a fighting chance of saving him with surgery. Buried in the daily swirl of more patients and even more surgery, I completely forgot about Mr. B for 2 months, until I saw his name on the clinic list again.

I steeled myself for the sight that I knew awaited me. Tumors that had burst forth from their confines, open malignant, evil sores, the sadness of the unrelenting pain that glazed the eyes. Above all, the smell of a combination of rotting flesh and tumors, that invaded your clothes, your skin, your nose and did not to let go for days.

"Hello Mr. B," I said, with the false jollity that we muster up in the worst of situations, as I stepped into his room.

Once again, I was shocked.

Not only did he not have any visible tumor, he actually had put on weight and looked tan and happy. Surely, this is not true; I remember thinking to myself, as we made small talk about his Cuba trip. Perhaps all the tumors were under the skin. They could not have all gone away with a single dose of the drug? Perhaps this was someone else? No, there was nothing to be found on my clinical exam or the follow-up CAT scan he got later in the day.

This is the closest thing to a medical miracle that I've ever witnessed, and it made me a believer.

I don't want you to think that everyone will have the response that Mr. B had when treated with these new drugs. While these drugs can seem miraculous in the desert of melanoma treatment, they are far from being the cure-all for the disease. Only a small number of people have the response that Mr. B did, and a slightly larger number will have a partial response. People who get these drugs can, and will, die of melanoma. There is still a lot more research to be done before we can treat all comers with melanoma and get the same miraculous results, but now, there is actually hope.

Back to the subject: How do these drugs actually work?

TARGETED THERAPY

Targeted therapy drugs attack cancer cells with less damage to regular cells. These drugs attack the particular harmful protein target in cancer cells.

The drugs we will talk about are Vemurafanib and Trametinib.

Let's start with <u>Vemurafanib</u> (commercial name Zelboraf). This drug was the first of the new group of drugs to be approved.

How is it taken? This pill is taken by mouth as prescribed by your doctor.

What makes Vemurafanib different? Vemurafanib is a chemical that is not produced by our body. Vemurafanib is given specifically to patients whose melanomas have the bad B-raf gene. The drug attacks the harmful B-raf protein produced by the tumors, not the gene itself, and kills it very quickly.

Why is that good? The normal cells are spared.

How does it work? This works differently than the other two drugs that we will talk about in the next section. Vemurafanib attacks a protein that is found only in melanoma cells. That protein is produced by a mutation in a gene called B-raf.

Remember: What you read in the earlier chapter and you will recall:

- Genes are a particular part of the DNA chain
- Genes are the instruction code that makes proteins in our bodies
- All of our normal cells have the B-raf gene
- Only the melanoma cells make the harmful B-raf protein, which helps the melanoma grow faster

That is why patients whose melanomas have the bad B-raf gene, are given Vemurafanib because it blocks the harmful B-raf protein and very quickly puts the brakes on cancer.

How do the Doctors know if the drug will or is working on the melanoma or not? The answer is through DNA testing. The doctors take a piece of the tumor tissue, then take the DNA out of the cells and analyze it for the mutation. It is paramount to remember, once again, it is the tumor alone that has the harmful B-raf gene and not the patient.

Isn't a blood test enough to tell? No. Testing the patient's blood will not give us useful information because the blood will be normal.

Is Vemurafanib a magic bullet? No. This seems like the perfect magic bullet; a drug that kills only the tumor cells and completely spares the healthy cells. However, real life is not that rosy. There are melanoma cells that do not have a mutant B-raf.

Does Vemurafanib affect all melanoma cells? As you can surmise, it is only the melanoma cells with the bad B-raf that will be affected by the drug. Therefore, all melanomas cannot be treated by Vemurafanib.

Does the body build up a resistance to Vemurafanib? Sometimes, the melanomas that initially responded to Vemurafanib develop resistance to the drug and the drug no longer kills the cells. These melanoma cells figure out a way of growing and spreading in ways that bypass the mutant B-raf gene. This could happen within a few months to a year of starting the drug. The result of resistance is that, even though the melanoma cells have the mutant gene, the drug no longer works.

Why use the drug in the first place if the tumors become resistant so soon? There are many reasons to use this drug. Since the drug is so effective, at least in the short term, it is extremely useful for treatment when there are tumors that are rapidly growing and are causing pain or discomfort to the patient. In the right patients, they can produce rapid relief.

Another good reason to use Vemurafanib is when there are tumors growing that cannot be treated by surgery.

Why Vemurafanib vs. surgery? Vemurafanib is also used when a patient has a number of sites in the body that have these tumors; such as the lung, skin, bone and abdomen. It may be possible to cut all of these tumors out surgically, but it's a very long and complicated surgery that could leave the patient mutilated. What is worse, in this kind of situation, the tumors can grow back at other sites, in a manner of weeks or months.

That's why treating this group of melanoma patients with Vemurafanib, rather than surgery, makes more sense.

Take home point: One of the more important aspects of treatment with Vemurafanib is that it buys the patient time so that he or she can be treated with the other two drugs (Ipi and Nivo) we are going to talk about later. This allows us to hit the melanoma with a one-two punch so that when it is trying to escape from the effects of Vemurafanib, it gets hit again.

What are Vemurafanib's possible side effects? Vemurafanib has many possible side effects that may include:

- Liver injury
- Severe skin reactions
- Sensitivity to the sun
- New skin cancers
- Alterations in heart rate or electric activity of the heart, especially in patients with prolonged QT syndrome

If you experience any of these out of the ordinary side effects, call your doctor and set up an appointment for a consultation.

Next, let's talk about **Trametinib** (commercial name Mekinist). Trametinib works on a different protein in the melanoma cell called MEK and is also a pill taken by mouth.

How does it work? Imagine two switches revving up the cancer in a kind of relay. MEK is a switch down the line from raf.

What makes it different? It targets regular MEK and not the mutated form.

Is Trametinib as effective as Vemurafinib? No, this drug is not as effective as Vemurafinib when used alone, but may be helpful if used in combination with Vemurafanib.

The immune system is one of the marvels of nature. Every organism has its version of the immune system to keep it healthy and fight invaders whether they are viruses, bacteria or fungi. The human immune system also recognizes cancer as an invader and launches a furious attack on it as soon as it is recognized. Cancers, and this includes melanomas, have figured out ways of escaping this attack, which is what makes them so lethal.

IMMUNOLOGY 101

To help explain how these drugs work we are going to take a detour. You can skip this section if you wish and move on to the next.

The cells in our blood that help us fight invaders are the white blood cells. The red blood cells carry oxygen and don't play a significant role in fighting invaders. Lymphocytes *(lim-fo sites)* are a type of white blood cell. There are two types. The T cells and the B cells, or T lymphocytes and B lymphocytes. The B cells make antibodies, a type of protein that help destroy invaders like bacteria. The T cells are like managers that help increase the number of B cells, the production of antibodies, and also increase their own numbers, i.e. produce more T cells. They do this by producing other special chemicals such as Interferon and Interleukin. These are the same chemicals that are used to fight melanoma.

The beauty of T cells is that they are very specific. Bacteria A will stimulate one type of T cell, and bacteria B will stimulate an entirely different type of T cell. The other important feature of T cells is they are trained not to attack our body. This is done in a variety of different ways including 'brakes' called CTLA4 and PDI. If these brakes were not present the T cells would start attacking the body's proteins, thinking that they were foreign proteins such as bacteria or viruses. The condition where the lymphocytes attack our bodies is called autoimmunity. This is a very harmful condition and can cause a lot of problems and may even lead to death.

What about the new drugs? The new drugs that we are going to talk–about are: **Ipilumimab**, which acts on one of the brakes of the T cells (CTLA4), **Nivolumab** (Nivo for short) and **Pembroluzimab** (Pembro for short), which acts on the second brake, PD1. The commercial names of these drugs are **Yervoy, Opdivo,** and **Keytruda** respectively.

How do the melanoma cells use these? They use them to escape the attack by the trained killer cells of our body. The major player, PD1, a protein, is like a lock on the surface of the T cells. The key to opening this lock is another protein called PD1 ligand or PDL1. The crafty melanoma cells produce a lot of PDL1 (the key) which then fits into the keyhole of the lock, the PD1 on the T cells, and turns off the T cells. The PD1 drugs, **Nivo** and **Pembro**, work by blocking the keyhole of the lock, as if someone put chewing gum on the keyhole of the lock so that the key does not fit. Unfortunately, the block only lasts for about a month, making the drug ineffective and the drug has to be given again.

How are these drugs administered? All these drugs are given intravenously. They cannot be given as a tablet since they would not be absorbed and more importantly, the digestive juices (including stomach acid) would destroy them since they are proteins.

Ipi works exactly the same way except that this gum blocks the lock CTLA4.

Then there are the Checkpoint Inhibitors—Ipilumimab, Nivolumimab, Pembrolumimab are also called checkpoint inhibitors. This title merely indicates how they work by removing or blocking the checkpoints or brakes.

Ipilumimab (also called Ipi) was the first drug of this class that was approved by the FDA in 2011. Its commercial name is Yervoy. The brake that Ipi works on is called CTLA4. This is an acronym for **C**ytotoxic **T** **L**ymphocyte **A**ntigen **4**. That is quite a mouthful, so let's stick with CTLA4. Nivolumab (also known as Nivo) and Pembrolizumab (Pembro for short), work to remove the brake on T lymphocytes (or T cells) called PD1. PD stands for **P**rogrammed **D**eath **1**.

Why not give all melanoma patients one of these drugs? The main problem is autoimmunity. This is a condition where the T cells attack our bodies. As a result of autoimmunity, you can get inflammation of the colon (colitis), lungs (pneumonitis), or the master endocrine gland—the pituitary (hypophysitis). Any of these conditions can be lethal. Therefore, one has to be very careful in giving these drugs to patients because the drugs themselves can kill the patient before cancer does. The drugs that act on PD1 (Nivo and Pembro) appear to have fewer side effects than those that act on CTLA4 (Ipi). This is one of the main reasons that patients that are receiving these drugs have to be monitored carefully.

What happens if you do get the symptoms of autoimmunity? It's simple; doctors can treat this in a variety of ways:

- They can reduce the dose of the drug or stop it altogether
- They can give steroids

In the case of severe colitis, they can give drugs such as Infliximab, which blunts the effects of inflammation in the colon or bowel.

What's the downside to these drugs? It takes a while for them to kick in. In some cases, the progress is so slow that it may take months to see progress. This slow progress has changed the way we now treat melanoma.

A decade ago if a tumor being treated by a drug increased in size, as seen on a CAT scan, it was always because the tumor was growing and not responding to therapy. However, with the new checkpoint drugs, an increase in the size of the tumor may mean that the body is responding by flooding in white blood cells to fight the cancer cells. This might make it seem like the tumor is growing when it actually is not.

Researchers soon realized that it would be possible to give both the PD1 inhibitors and the CTLA4 inhibitors together. This improved the effects of treatment since they targeted different brakes. They also reasoned that they could give lower doses and minimize the side effects of both the drugs. The first result of these trials was published last year and proved to be among the most spectacular results ever obtained in the treatment of melanoma. This was particularly important for me as some of my patients were a part of this trial and were among those who benefited from it.

For example: Let's say Mr. Jones comes with large tumors of his groin, neck, and lungs. He also has tumors that involve his spine and is in constant agony from the pain of the cancer in his bones. He has a mutant B-raf in his tumors.

What might be the best way to treat him? Based on what we have discussed, an excellent way to treat him might be to start him on Vemurafanib. Once he begins to respond and is not so sick, he can be started on a combination of Nivo and Ipi. The logic of this treatment is that Mr. Jones can get rapid relief of his pain through Vemurafanib as well as control of the size of his tumors. Once he starts to improve, his immune system will also recover. At this point, we can release the brakes and unleash his immune system to fight his tumors. One of the advantages of starting the Vemurfanib first is that the tumors get smaller, so the immune system can theoretically work its magic better since the enemy is smaller. The truly amazing feature of this scenario is that we have not once discussed surgery as an option. That's the miracle of what research can do for cancer patients.

What About Experimental Therapies?

What if the so-called miracle treatments don't work and the melanoma still continues to grow and spread? Is that the end of the road?

The answer is a resounding NO!

If a patient is at this point the decision to seek further treatment or opt for hospice care becomes a very personal and philosophical one. The important thing is to realize that there is no right answer. Since the basic premise underlying this book is **HOPE**, this part of the book is for those patients who wish to soldier on.

ADOPTIVE CELL TRANSFER

The key player in organizing the attack on melanomas is the T cell or T lymphocyte. Because these cells are crippled for various reasons in melanoma patients they are not able to mount a response to destroy the cancer cells. In this case, melanoma cells.

Previously, we discussed how the new drugs can remove the brakes and let the T cells fight again. Another approach was devised where the T cells attacking the tumor were removed by cutting out some of the tumor and then grown in the laboratory, acting in part as a sort of T cell farm. The T cells removed from the tumors are called TILs, (**T**umor **I**nfiltrating **L**ymphocytes). Millions of these T cells are grown and then given intravenously back to the patient where the thought was/is they would/will destroy the tumors. Sometimes Interleukin-2 (IL-2) is also given simultaneously to make these T cells grow—a sort of T cell fertilizer. Researchers at The National Institute of Health found that the only way to make these millions of new cells survive in the body was to get rid of the old ones, either through chemotherapy or radiation. As you can imagine, this is a very involved and toxic process. The logic of this method is that unless you remove a house of its old tenants it is impossible to bring in the new owners who can start their families.

The interval where the old white cells are destroyed, and the new ones are introduced is a very vulnerable time for the patients since they can be very prone to infections. Therefore, they are very carefully monitored and treated as the situation demands.

Some of the unique side effects of this treatment is the so-called *cytokine storm* or the *tumor lysis syndrome*. As this treatment involves administering a large number of fighting T cells, a vast amount of the tumor may be killed in a very short time releasing massive quantities of various chemicals. The body may not be able to cope with these chemicals, called cytokines, and may even result in the death of the patient.

Are all melanoma patients candidates for radiation?
No, not all patients are candidates for this treatment for various reasons such as:

- There might not be enough tumor to harvest the TILs
- The harvested TILs may refuse to grow in the "farm" for unknown reasons
- The patient may be medically too sick to undergo a very strenuous treatment course like those outlined

Is there anything else we can do? What else can be done? What other treatments can be used? There are other ingenious treatments such as TCR (T cell Receptor Therapy) and CAR (Chimeric Antigen Therapy) being tried out in metastatic melanoma with some success.

WHAT ABOUT VACCINATIONS?

The thought of using the body's immune system to fight melanoma is not new. One of the longest known methods in use is the injection of proteins, specific to melanomas, into the patient's body so as to coax the cells to fight the tumor. This is exactly the same principle we use when we get our annual flu shot. This has not been as successful because we don't know the exact protein, or proteins that will do the trick. The tumors have a way of crippling these T cells even if they were able to mount a response.

ARE COMBINATION TREATMENTS AN OPTION?

Any of these treatments can be used in combination. For instance, doctors in Boston have combined the use of the checkpoint inhibitors with a drug that stimulates the bone marrow cells to multiply. The thought behind this is that once the brakes are removed, and the T cells are free to grow, why not help them develop more by adding a fertilizer into the body itself? Other groups have used radiation in combination with checkpoint inhibitors with the thought that radiation can create more bits of tumor which can be recognized by the T cells and can mount a better attack. There is also another group that has proposed using a vaccination in combination with the checkpoint inhibitors.

WHAT IS A CLINICAL TRIAL?

A clinical trial is a carefully regulated experiment to see if one method of treating a disease is better than another.

Are these trials regulated? Yes, these experiments have to be approved by a committee that oversees research in human beings and are not allowed to move forward until this approval is obtained. Any side effects from a new drug are very carefully monitored by the physicians running the study. A study may involve the comparison of a new drug against a well-established treatment. The reason a study is done is because the doctors do not know if the new drug is better (or worse) than the other drugs they are using. There is no way of finding this out in real life other than trying it out on patients.

If you're considering a clinical trial, it's important that you ask questions and weigh the pros and cons for your life and situation.

How do you find a clinical trial that's right for you? To learn more about clinical trials, talk to your cancer team.

Here are the questions to help you decide what is right for you.

- What clinical trial is best for me? Why?

- What happens if I decide not to do a clinical trial?
- What will happen to me without the new treatment?
- What are my other treatment choices?
- Will I know which treatment I receive?
- What are the side effects and how severe or likely are they?
- Will the study cost me anything or is treatment free?
- If I'm harmed as a result of the research, what treatment am I entitled?
- Will I have to stay in the hospital during the study?
- Will there be a long-term follow-up?
- Has this treatment been used to treat other cancers?

The American Cancer Society offers a clinical trial matching service that will help you decide which trial, if any, may be right for you: http://clinicaltrials.cancer.org or by calling 1-800-303-5691.

WARNING! Patients who have widespread disease, rapidly growing disease or disease that does not respond to treatment are placed in a very difficult position. We all have a natural tendency to seek alternative treatments that are unproven and are often unsafe. The Internet has made matters worse since there is so much unedited information that is so easily available. The biggest danger is that patients may seek these unproven treatments over those which are experimental but carefully monitored, thus missing out on a potential advantage. It's most important to stay safe when we are feeling desperate and to trust your care providers who will safely guide you on your journey through these uncharted territories.

SEVEN

RADIATION FOR MELANOMA

Radiation and melanomas were thought to be incompatible for the longest time. This was the result of a concept called *radioresistance* where the melanoma metastases were believed to harbor an inbuilt defense against radiation. Recent research has shown that by changing the dose and the frequency at which radiation is given doctors can make good use of radiation in the treatment of this problem. You must know that there is a grain of truth to the radioresistance concept, in that the melanomas don't melt away in the face of radiation like other tumors do.

Therefore, the bottom line is that when used appropriately, radiation is extremely effective in cases of metastatic melanoma.

The most significant use of radiation in melanomas is for the treatment of brain metastases. The so-called "Gamma knife" allows for the precision treatment of metastases located in most parts of the brain, including many that are inaccessible to surgeons. The use of this treatment has significantly prolonged the lives of many patients with melanoma metastases to the brain. Even more encouraging is the fact that unlike the past years (given appropriately sized and located tumors), up to 20 tumors can be treated. This is a great advance in the treatment of this problem because the previous treatment, called "whole brain radiation," was not as effective and left the patient with significant side effects. Gamma knife treatment is used in specialized centers and involves the combined expertise of a neurosurgeon, a radiation oncologist (a doctor who uses X-rays to treat medical problems) and a radiation physicist to precisely calculate the dose and treatment needed to provide the maximal benefit.

This concept of precision bombing of melanoma metastases can also be used in areas that are difficult to get to surgically such as behind the breastbone, close to the heart.

Another scenario where radiation is used in melanoma is metastases to the bone. In this scenario, it may be a huge deal to cut out the bone that has a tumor. Radiation can take care of this in a much less invasive fashion. Radiating the bony metastases can help relieve the pain, which is a common symptom of this problem.

There has been a recent trend to use radiation in an effort to prevent local recurrence after a node dissection in the axilla. The concern is that this has not been shown to improve survival rates should the melanoma return at that site. It becomes very difficult for the surgeon to offer any options because of the difficulty in operating in a radiated field. The difficulty results from the fact that radiation produces a lot of scarring so operating in the area is akin to hacking through concrete. Additionally, wounds in a radiated area tend to heal very slowly.

Thus, a recurrence in a site after radiation is a very unpleasant situation.

EIGHT

EXPERIMENTAL THERAPIES

CLINICAL TRIALS

A clinical trial is a carefully regulated experiment to see if one method of treating a disease is better than another. These experiments have to be approved by a committee that oversees research in human beings and are not allowed to move forward until this approval is obtained. Any side effects from a new drug are very carefully monitored by the physicians running the study. A study may involve the comparison of a new drug against a well-established treatment.

The reason a study is done is because the doctors do not know if the new drug is better (or worse) than the other drugs they are using. There is no better way of finding this out in real life than trying it out on patients.

If you're considering a clinical trial, it's important that you ask questions and weigh the pros and cons for your life and situation. To find out more about clinical trials, talk to your cancer team. You may want to ask the following questions to get a clearer picture:

- What clinical trial is best for me? And why?
- What happens if I decide not to do a clinical trial? What will happen to me without the new treatment?
- What are my other treatment choices?
- Will I know which treatment I receive?
- What are the side effects, and how severe or likely are they?
- Will the study cost me anything, or is treatment free?
- If I'm harmed as a result of the research, what treatment am I entitled?
- Will I have to stay in the hospital during the study?
- Will there be a long-term follow-up?
- Has the treatment been used to treat other cancers?

The American Cancer Society offers a clinical trial matching service that will help you decide which trial may be right for you: http://clinicaltrials.cancer.org or by calling 1-800-303-5691.

FROM SURVIVOR
TO THRIVER

NINE

LIFESTYLE STEPS

If you have been diagnosed with melanoma or any cancer for that matter, you know firsthand how hard it is to stay positive and remain hopeful. The big fight isn't the fight against cancer. The big fight is the war that is going on in our heads, every minute of every day. Our minds can become our worst enemy. Keeping an optimistic outlook is the single most important thing you need to do to win this fight. Not to keep cancer away but more importantly, not to allow cancer to tell you who you are.

In fact, staying positive is essential when it comes to healing. Countless studies show that people who reject depression and despair have a better chance of being cured. That's right. You can dismiss the negative thoughts. In fact, your life depends on it.

How do you remain confident when you hear the worst possible news that changes your life in an instant? How do you stay optimistic when you don't feel well and your friends are out having fun while you are going to doctor appointment after doctor appointment?

It takes a team to win this fight, and right now your body needs you in the boxing ring to fight the most important fight of your life.

Are You Ready? You may feel helpless in this struggle against cancer, but the truth is there is a lot you can do to feel better physically, mentally and spiritually—right now. One of the most frustrating things is that you can't go back and change what you did growing up. You certainly can't change your genetic make-up that sets you up any more than you can change the color of your eyes. However, you do get to decide how you fight back—now, today. There are ways you can lower your risk for future disease and make sure your family is fighting the good fight and boosting your immunity, following these three simple steps.

1. Eating a healthy diet
2. Exercising and moving daily
3. Positive outlook | Spiritual belief

Number three is where most people fall because it's unseen, or is it? We go to the doctors when we are physically ill, but what do we do when our heart hurts, or we are scared and anxious? How do we protect our spiritual body? After all we are spiritual beings, having human experiences, not the other way around. But how do we get our whole body in agreement to fight and win?

Your entire body needs to be in the ring for this battle and even doctors agree that people who believe (and have a positive outlook) seem to deal with their disease better than those who don't. One of the problems I have with all of this *spiritual* stuff is that when I'm sick and not feeling well, my body shuts down. Not just physically, but emotionally. I shut off from people who love me, which means I shut off my support systems inside and outside. That makes me exactly the kind of person cancer likes to attack. It's crucial to step out of your safe zone and fight the battle of your life, for your life, and WIN.

Cancer may have a one-two punch, but you can beat it because you can fight back with 1, 2, 3 knockout punches. Are you ready to fight?

EATING A HEALTHY DIET: SIX HEALTH HABITS THAT BOOST AND KEEP YOU STRONG

A healthy and active functioning immune system does play a role in maintaining the body's resistance to melanomas.

> **YOU MUST KNOW** that a diet alone cannot cure melanoma

One of the best ways to boost your immune system, and feel better fast, is to fuel your body with clean food. Eating an organic whole foods diet, and drinking plenty of pure water, is the best way to support your immune system so it can fight off cancer and prevent recurrence. The foods discussed here are of particular importance for their cancer-fighting properties.

This isn't about depriving yourself, or jumping on the crazy diet schemes that are promising to rid your body of cancer. Rather, it's a new way of life to keep your body strong and healthy. Focus on what you can eat versus what you can't. Eating clean 80 percent of the time allows you a 20 percent margin for eating the foods you love. As long as you are 80/20, you're doing more than enough to keep yourself healthy.

Perfection does not exist, and we are all human. Be gentle with yourself and allow yourself a special treat as long as you have nourished your body with the nutrients it needs by eating clean, pure foods. In other words, good enough is good enough.

Health Habit #1: If it's White, it's Not Right

Avoid refined carbohydrates. Refined carbohydrates are high on the glycemic index, and raise blood sugar levels which promotes fat storage, increases appetite, promotes certain cancers and increases rapid fluctuations in blood sugar that aggravates brain function. All of these make you feel weak and tired. Remember, if it's "white", it's not right for your body.

The "White's" that should be blacklisted:

- Potatoes
- Pasta
- Rice
- All white flour products including bagels, granola, instant oatmeal, muffins, potato chips, pastries, pretzels. All bread, including rye, pumpernickel and gourmet bread, tortilla chips, all cereal bars, and crackers—unless listed on the approved list.

Did you know that sushi contains refined rice? Prepackaged products contain processed refined carbohydrates. These foods are high on the glycemic index, high in fat, and low in fiber. They do not provide the nourishment your body needs. They rob and deplete your body instead. They are high in trans fatty acids to give them a long shelf life. Instead choose foods that are on the Good-For-You-Grains list.

Lastly, remember the stress factor. Too much restriction in your diet can cause stress, so if you love macaroni and cheese, then have a small portion once in a while. There is no "good" stress.

Health Habit #2: Go for Good-for-You-Grains

Grains provide necessary vitamins; especially B vitamins, phytochemicals, and minerals. They are full of fiber, which blunts blood sugar release. You and your body need grains for energy unless you're overweight or diabetic. In that case, you should follow your doctor's orders when it comes to eating carbohydrates.

While pasta, bread, and cereals (including cereal bars), can raise blood sugar levels, there are higher quality whole grains that can help you avoid this. Most prepackaged foods contain refined carbohydrates. It's better to eat from the earth, meaning choose foods that are not processed and are as close to their natural state as possible.

Not sure if food is processed or packaged? Think—can I pick it? If you can pick it, you can eat it. Foods like sweet potatoes, brown rice, and whole oats are not processed. This means they are mostly natural without sugar added, compared to cereals, bread, and other packaged convenience foods.

Go-To Good-For-You-Grains

- All Bran
- Oat Bran
- Oatmeal (not instant)
- Uncle Sam dry cereal
- Whole wheat pancakes and waffles
- Barley
- Brown rice
- Buckwheat
- Spinach or chickpea pasta
- Wasa crackers
- Vita Wheat Crisp
- Whole wheat and whole grain bread (must contain at least 3 grams of fiber)
- Whole wheat tortilla
- Quinoa

WARNING: Just because the food says it's healthy on the label, doesn't mean it is. Labels can be very deceiving. Read the label and look for sugar, carbohydrates and lack of fiber to distinguish a Good-For-You-Grain from a horrible health food.

Look for the word "whole" in front of the grain in the ingredients when purchasing your food products, to be sure you're not getting the refined version. Regularly eating whole grains will help you stay healthy and keep energy levels balanced all day. At the same time, you will be lowering your cholesterol and blood pressure. This will help stabilize blood glucose and insulin levels while reducing heart disease, stroke, diabetes and protecting you from certain cancers.

Good-For-You-Grains are especially important during and after treatments to help prevent and deal with side effects such as IBS and diverticulitis while keeping you regular.

HEALTH HABIT #3: POWER UP YOUR IMMUNITY WITH VEGETABLES AND *SOME* FRUIT

Load up on vegetables and *some* fruit. They are nutrient powerhouses that make them the best carbohydrate choices. They add variety and flavor to your diet and provide fiber, vitamins, phyto-nutrients, and antioxidants.

Vegetables: This food group is by far the most overlooked food group and most people do not meet their daily requirement of them. Vegetables play a crucial role in the healing process because they keep our bodies alkaline in check while helping reduce inflammation, which may speed healing and reduce pain.

Vegetables should be lightly cooked vs. raw or overcooked for better nutrient absorption. Fresh is best and frozen is fine, but limit canned vegetables if you can. Fruit also contributes to a variety of vitamins and minerals, but fruit can also raise blood sugar levels, which may lead to an energy crash.

While no one vegetable is going to cure cancer, you should be aware that vegetables are the best source of all nutrients, and should be your first choice, making fruit a second option. There are certain vegetables that are superior to others. They will be starred (*) on the vegetable list.

Aim to eat five ½ cup servings of vegetables and two ½ cup servings of fruit daily. If weight is not an issue, have as much fruit as desired. Dried fruits such as raisins, dates, and apricots should be avoided or limited, as they are high in sugar and lower in nutrition. Choose powerhouse fruits as much as possible.

DID YOU KNOW?

Fruit raises blood sugar the same way candy does. It's okay if you're suffering with blood sugar crash after you treatments; however, you should always try to have some protein or a small serving of nuts along with it to help stabilize sugar swings.

Cancer-Fighting Compounds: Vegetables in the cruciferous family (marked with an asterisk) contain indoles. Indoles are compounds that act as detoxifying agents. Indoles are believed to remove cancer-causing substances from the body.

Powerhouse Vegetables and Fruits to Choose: The serving size of green leafy vegetables is 1 cup or the size of your fist. The serving size of all others is a ½ cup or the size of a light bulb—primarily raw vegetables and vegetables used for juicing.

Fruits are not necessary, so there isn't a suggested serving size, but it's helpful to satisfy your sweet tooth naturally. Stick to one to two ½ cup servings daily. A ½ cup is equivalent to a tennis ball.

Vegetables: (* vegetables are superior to others)

- Artichoke hearts
- Arugula

- Asparagus
- Bamboo shoots
- Beans (green, wax, Italian)
- Broccoli*
- Brussel sprouts*
- Cabbage * (red, green, purple, Chinese)
- Carrots
- Cauliflower*
- Celery
- Chives
- Collards*
- Cucumber
- Eggplant
- Endive
- Garlic
- Kale*
- Kohlrabi
- Leeks
- Lettuce (except iceberg) and micro greens
- Mushrooms (look for Enoki mushrooms)*
- Mustard greens*
- Okra
- Onions
- Peppers
- Seaweed
- Snow peas
- Spinach
- Squash (zucchini, summer, yellow, spaghetti)
- Turnips
- Water chestnut
- Watercress

If blood sugar swings are an issue for you, limit carrots, tomatoes, beets, corn, and pumpkin.

Fruit:

- Apples
- Applesauce (unsweetened)
- Apricots
- Berries (limit strawberries)
- Cantaloupe
- Cherries
- Figs
- Grapefruit
- Guava
- Honeydew melons
- Kiwifruit
- Lychees
- Mandarin orange
- Mangoes
- Nectarines
- Oranges
- Papayas
- Peaches
- Pears
- Pineapples
- Plums

You may want to limit the sweeter fruits due to their sugar content and GI response.

Examples: Bananas, mangoes, papaya, pineapple, as well as the very high dried fruits like raisins, strawberries, watermelon, dates, etc. (except dried apricots). Canned fruits packed in heavy syrup, and fruit found in yogurts are extremely high in sugar and don't count towards your daily nutrient quota.

HEALTH HABIT #4: POWER UP YOUR IMMUNITY WITH THE RIGHT PROTEIN

Protein Power: We need protein in our diet to get the vitamins and minerals required for healing and optimal health. Protein is king when it comes to boosting our immunity and healing after medical procedures.

Protein helps to stabilize blood sugar levels and blunt insulin response when combined with high sugar or carb-filled foods and can help keep us feeling fuller, longer. Balancing blood sugar levels can become difficult after receiving treatments, so the suggestions made here need to become a way of life.

> **If you're a vegetarian, there are many alternatives for getting the proper amount of protein and minerals you would normally get from eating meat and fish. Since healing and recovery place increased demands on our bodies it's important that you pay very close attention to your nutrient requirements, and you should seek help while you're healing.**
>
> **This problem is easily solved by drinking a whey protein shake every day, or having egg whites and consuming some fish, which are better options than trying to get your nutrient needs from tofu and dairy.**

While meat is a good source of protein and iron, not all proteins are created equal. Meat is also a source of saturated fat and cholesterol. Choosing the right kind makes all the difference in the world when it comes to health and healing.

Fish is an excellent source of protein because it contains Omega-3 fatty acids, but can be a source of mercury, as well as contain organic pollutants such as PCBs.

The *incredible edible egg* is almost perfect and full of nutrients, so you should eat whole eggs in moderation.

Milk, cheese, and other dairy products are made from animal fat. They should be eaten in moderation (but they do provide some protein and calcium essential to our health). Treat dairy as a dessert and enjoy some each day, keeping your health budget in the 80/20 guidelines. Dairy falls in the 20 percent category.

Trying to find the right balance of protein is critical when we are recovering, and isn't always easy. Too much protein can lead to calcium and bone loss because it creates high phosphate levels. This may be an issue for anyone with impaired kidney function because it limits their ability to handle the nitrogen load found in protein.

I suggest that you have a clean whey protein shake every day to ensure that your body gets the nutrition it needs without all of the saturated fat and cholesterol. Protein shakes make it easy, and save you money in the long run.

Aim to have a small portion of protein the size of a deck of cards with each meal. If you're feeling too sick to eat, supplement with a protein shake. They are easier on your stomach and digest very quickly, so your body gets a hit of the nutrition it needs helping you to feel better, faster.

Poultry: Serving size is 3 ounces cooked

- Chicken breast
- Turkey breast
- Cornish hens

Why not the leg? Legs are higher in iron and zinc, which are good for healing, but legs contain more saturated fat. You should limit them to once a week. Yes, even if you're trying to gain weight. You never want to gain weight at the expense of your health.

Meat in moderation. Limit to one serving per week. A serving is 4 ounces uncooked, which shrinks to 3 ounces cooked. Even if you're trying to gain weight, the proteins listed in this section need to be limited.

Beef:

- Round steak
- Sirloin tip
- Lean ground meat only (look for at least 95 percent lean or no more than 10 grams of fat, per 3 ounce serving)

Lamb:

- Leg
- Loin
- Shank

Minimize these meats:

- Fatty marbled and prime cut meat or hamburger
- Lamb: Ground or mutton, which is the meat of an adult lamb (older equals more risk of pesticides, growth hormones, etc.)

What about Pork? Avoid it. It's not the other white meat. Not only is it an inferior source of protein, but it's also high in fat and cholesterol. Pork has been known to carry a variety of toxic substances and pathogens. That is the last thing your body needs right now when you are trying to boost immunity. Sacrificing a little taste is worth not sacrificing your health.

Avoid:

- Bacon
- Ham hocks
- Pigs feet
- Spare ribs
- Short ribs
- Pork sausages

When It Comes To Meats, Here Is What and How You Should Eat It:

- Organic and grass fed meat is recommended, whenever possible
- Meat that has been cooked healthfully by braising, roasting and broiling
- Skin poultry and trim fat from all meats before cooking
- Make stews and soups ahead of time and refrigerate them. Once they are cooled, remove the fat that you can see from the top before you reheat the dish.
- When making casseroles or meat sauces, brown the meat first, and then discard the fat before adding other ingredients. **Note:** *This may seem counter-intuitive if you're trying to gain weight. Not only is this fat toxic and harmful to your body, but it also prevents you from being hungry, often enough to satisfy your bodies nutritional needs.*

Meats and Things You Shouldn't Eat:

- Limit consumption of unhealthy proteins, such as lunchmeats
- Avoid grilled meats, as they generate high levels of carcinogens
- Never cook meat with butter or solid margarine (they are extremely high in hydrogenated fats and are very rough on the stomach)

Fascinating Fish Facts: Fish is one of the best sources of protein because it's low in fat and high in Omega-3 fatty acids. It's important to choose the right kind of fish, or you'll end up with mercury and pesticides, which may affect your immune system. Only choose the fish listed here, and aim to eat fish daily, if possible. The Omega-3 fatty acids found in fish are miraculous when it comes to boosting immunity and promoting healing.

Eat all you want of these types of fish. They are lowest in mercury levels:

- Catfish
- Clams
- Salmon (Pacific)
- Tilapia
- Shrimp
- Anchovies
- Flounder
- Haddock
- Sardines
- Scallops
- Sole (Pacific)
- Squid (calamari)
- Trout (fresh water)
- Whitefish

Moderate Mercury Level Fish: Eat these types of fish moderately, as they fall into the medium mercury level group. Eat them once a week. Pregnant women in their reproductive years should limit eating them to once a month.

- Mahi-Mahi
- Snapper
- Bass
- Cod
- Halibut
- Lobster

High Mercury Level Fish: It's best to avoid these fish altogether, as a single serving can put you over the EPA (Environmental Protection Agency) safe limit for the month. Your immune system doesn't need anymore to deal with.

- Bluefish
- Chilean Sea Bass
- Grouper
- Orange Roughy
- Shark

- Swordfish
- Tuna (canned, Albacore, Ahi, Yellowfin)
- Mackerel

Did you know that mercury causes the immune system to malfunction? Not the best idea when trying to boost immunity.

Free For All Fish Facts:

- If you see it listed, it's ok to eat
- Frozen fish is fine if it's flash frozen
- Wild caught, or line caught fish is the best kind to eat for immune boosting
- Cook your fish by baking or poaching for healthy results

DID YOU KNOW?

It's the food that fish are fed or eat that leads to high PCB levels, not the water the fish swim in. The higher the fat level of the fish, the more contaminants, as fat is where they are stored.

Fish and Cooking Techniques:

- Canned tuna is too high in PCBs and should be limited
- Remove skin to remove fat from fish, and reduce PCB risk
- Do not fry fish. It defeats the purpose because it destroys the nutrients.
- The lighter the meat of the fish, the better it is for you
- Some shellfish such as shrimp and lobster, as well as caviar, are high in cholesterol. They are safe to eat in limited amounts. *Monthly equals Moderation.*

DID YOU KNOW?

By eating 2 cans of tuna you can ingest 35 micrograms of mercury, exceeding the 38.5 microgram weekly limit. The National Academy of Sciences and the EPA set PCB assessment and consumption limits. Unfortunately, fish with the lowest mercury levels don't always have the highest Omega-3 levels. Supplementing with a high-quality Omega-3 is a very good idea. This is the one way to guarantee that your body gets the right amount of DHA and EPA (fatty acids) needed to boost immunity.

Look for an Omega-3 that contains the right amount of DHA and EPA, which is 500 milligrams of each. Remember you get what you pay for, and in this department it's worth it to spend a little more to get an excellent Omega-3 supplement.

This class of fat plays a critical role in immune boosting and easing inflammation, which is critical when we are healing from procedures, and to help offset side effects.

> **LET YOUR DOCTOR KNOW** that you are taking Omega-3 supplements, and be sure to stop taking them at least 10 days before surgery to avoid complications!

Incredible Eggs: Eggs are a nutritional powerhouse. The high cholesterol content of yolks has given them a bad rap. However, this may not be entirely accurate as shown by more recent research. Until this situation is clarified, it may be a good idea to limit consumption to three eggs a week if you insist on eating the whole egg.

If you have elevated cholesterol, are being treated for it or are at high risk for heart disease, ask your doctor for his input or limit yourself to the egg whites. The white of the egg is the part that contains the protein. In removing the yolk, you still get most if not all the benefits, without the drawbacks. It's best to stick to the egg whites when you're recovering from radiation or other treatment therapies because your body digests and utilizes the nutrients better, as yolks are harder to digest.

Keep in mind that a lot of the foods we eat contain eggs such as baked goods, pancakes, as well as sauces and dressings. Try to stick to fresh eggs and remove the yolks yourself. Eggbeaters are also okay in moderation.

Fresh is always best. Egg whites are delicious. Get creative by adding vegetables or salmon for a quick, satisfying meal. Egg white omelets are an excellent choice when eating out and can be found anywhere, at any time these days.

> **AVOID** preparing eggs with butter, milk or cheese. Save those heavy choices for treat days.

HEALTH HABIT #5: POWER FATS FOR A POWERFUL IMMUNE SYSTEM

The fact is we all need fat. Every cell in our body requires fat. Fats help nutrient absorption, nerve cell transmissions and contribute to protecting cell integrity. In fact, some fats are needed for cancer drugs to work better.

While some fats are good for you, most are not, and can clog our arteries and cause inflammation and do other damage. Most people don't understand the difference between good fats and bad fats or how much we need each day to stay healthy. Not all fats are created equal, and the best way to protect your health is to replace the bad fats with good-for-you fats.

Fat Facts You Need To Know: Good Fats—Monounsaturated Fats (or MUFAS) help lower total cholesterol and LDL (bad cholesterol), while increasing HDL cholesterol (the good cholesterol). MUFAS also have been known to reduce cancer risk, as well as overall mortality.

Olive oil is one of the best-tasting, good-for-you monounsaturated fats. Extra virgin olive oil is loaded with polyphenols that are essential antioxidants with heart benefits.

Spanish olive oils are known for having the highest level of hydroxytyrosol, which is a very potent antioxidant that helps reduce inflammation, and counteracts oxidative stress. There are many MUFAS that are good for you including nuts and avocados, but before you take that first bite, you should check out the complete list provided.

Poly Unsaturated Fats: Called essential fats because the body may not be able to synthesize them, or make them.

This group of fats also lowers cholesterol and LDL cholesterol. Omega-3 fats belong to this group of good-for-you fats. Some of these are seafood like salmon; as well as fish oil, soy, corn, flax, safflower and sunflower oils.

Polyunsaturated fats are more important than you think. These VIP fats are essential because they are crucial for growth, health and healthy cellular function.

What You Might Not Know About Good Fats Might Hurt Your Health: By not eating enough of the good-for-you fats, and eating too much of the bad fats, you create the perfect storm for disease.

Almost 90 percent of us consume excessive amounts of Omega-6 and don't eat enough Omega-3 every day. Omega-6 has been linked to diseases such as diabetes and certain cancers. It is also popular in fad diets such as Paleo, Atkins, South Beach and Mediterranean.

Our Western (or American diet) is full of processed and refined foods that contain excessive amounts of Omega-6, yet are severely lacking in Omega-3. This creates an imbalance, which sets us up for disease. Our diets should be a 4:1 ratio—4 parts Omega-3 to 1 part Omega-6. We consume a 15:1 ratio in a typical American diet. This is bad for our health.

Both Omega-6 and Omega-3 are metabolized similarly in the body because their molecular structure is similar. They also compete for many of the same enzymes. However, there is a catch. Once they hook up with an enzyme, they behave very differently.

The molecules that arise when Omega-3's are metabolized provide a whole host of potential anti-cancer benefits. They show the ability to reduce the production of other cancer-promoting enzymes, increase the rate at which cancer cells die, and may help prevent other cancer cells from forming. At the same time, preventing blood vessel formation needed for them to grow, also known as angiogenesis.

On the other hand when Omega-6 pairs up with an enzyme, the resulting molecule can promote inflammation, and cause cells to multiply and decrease cancer cell death. This is precisely what you don't want.

There is a role for Omega-6 fats, but when they are consumed out of proportion they cut off the protective benefits of Omega-3 fats. Avoiding the use of corn oil based products and using more canola oil instead adjusts an out of balance, harmful ratio.

Where Are Omega-6 Fats Found? Omega-6 oils are found in vegetable oils such as corn oil, safflower, sunflower, and soybean. These oils are also used in processed snacks, baked goods, and commercial salad dressings.

Omega-3 Fats Are Hiding Here: Omega-3 fats are found mostly in fish like salmon, sardines, trout, and herring. Omega-3 is also present, but in smaller amounts, in canola oil, flaxseed, green leafy vegetables (another good reason to eat your veggies), and walnuts.

The best choices of seafood are cold-water fish.

The best plant sources are flaxseed and flaxseed oil, canola oil, walnuts, wheat germ, and green leafy vegetables such as spinach, kale, leeks, and broccoli.

What's The Big Risk? We have known for some time that when omega fats are balanced, the risk for most cancers such as prostate, breast and colon cancers is lower.

What you may not know is that your risk for inflammatory conditions such as arthritis is also reduced. Omega-3 fats contribute to health by improving nutritional status, which may help host immunity. It has also shown promise for patients with advanced cancer, and in some cases contributes to longer survival rates.

Omega-3 also has a reputation for possibly helping cancer drugs work more efficiently, and may also help reduce side effects from treatment. Research is looking at the possibility of Omega-3's reducing tumor growth.

Let's face it, when we eat healthy fats, it not only tastes great, it's satisfying and helps keep us feeling full with little or no insulin response. Regularly consuming these good-for-you fats is the single most important dietary strategy to protect your health.

Consume the majority of your fat calories from the monounsaturated varieties, as these provide powerful cardiovascular protection:

- Extra virgin olive oil
- Expeller pressed canola oil
- Nuts/seeds
- Avocados

Make an extra effort to have at least one serving of Omega-3 fats every day:

- Oily fish (salmon, tuna, mackerel, sardines, herring, lake trout, etc., are the richest sources)
- Walnuts
- Canola oil
- Flaxseed
- Omega-3 eggs
- Dark leafy greens

Omega-3 fat benefits the cardiovascular system. They also play a critical role in proper brain function, aids in controlling excessive inflammation in the body and boosts immunity.

Avoid trans fats such as stick margarine, shortening, and products containing hydrogenated and partially hydrogenated oils.

Trans fats are horrible for your cardiovascular system, because they increase bad cholesterol (LDL), increase triglycerides, as well as reduce blood clotting while decreasing good cholesterol (HDL). Trans fats also increase insulin resistance, which predisposes us to weight gain.

Minimize these saturated fats:

- Fatty cuts of beef, pork, and lamb

- Whole dairy products (whole milk, cream, ice cream, cheese)

Like trans fats, saturated fat elevates your cholesterol, increases your chances of heart disease, and increases your insulin resistance.

Good-For-You Fats:

- Almonds
- Canola oil
- Cashews
- Mayonnaise made with canola oil
- Olive oil
- Peanuts
- Peanut butter (avoid peanut butter made with trans fats and make sure it's organic)
- Pecans
- Reduced-fat salad dressing
- Soft tub margarine labeled no TFA (made with 50 percent vegetable oil)
- Walnuts

Not Good-For-You Fats:

- Butter
- Cheese
- Corn oil
- Lard
- Margarine
- Stick
- Mayonnaise (most commercial brands)
- Peanut butter (unless it's organic)
- Peanut oil sauces
- Salad dressings (commercial)
- Shortening (hard)
- Side bacon
- Suet
- Trans fatty acids

HEALTH HABIT #6: GO NUTS!

Have a moderate handful (1 ounce) every day, in place of processed snacks. These nutrient powerhouses are not only good for weight loss but also one of the most heart-healthy foods you can eat.

Multiple studies show that as little as 1 ounce of nuts, 5 times weekly, can reduce cardiovascular risk by 30-50 percent. Their trio of vegetable protein, fiber, and healthy fat provide a powerful ally in your health betterment efforts. They can also aid in weight loss efforts.

Best Choices:

- Walnuts
- Almonds
- Cashews
- Pistachios
- Hazelnuts
- Brazil nuts
- Pecans
- Pine nuts
- Flax seeds
- Sunflower seeds
- Sesame seeds

Did you now that Brazil nuts contain more selenium than any other food and is thought to be one of the most potent immune systems boosters and antioxidants? This may sound beneficial; however, the amount of selenium is so high that eating them too frequently puts you at risk of selenium toxicity. As long as you eat only a few, Brazil nuts are a good source of magnesium, vitamin E, and healthy unsaturated fats.

> **The best way to ensure that you get the proper amount of Omega-3 is to supplement with a pharmaceutical-grade Omega-3 supplement.**

TEN

Exercising and Moving Daily

Exercise is THE Best Medicine

Science shows the single best thing you can do for your physical and emotional health and recovery is (drum roll)—exercise. That means no matter how sick you are, or how much you weigh, the best thing you can do is start moving.

Exercise helps prevent and improve just about any condition or ailment you're struggling to handle. From pain reduction, immunity boosting, depression, fatigue, water retention to appetite regulation. Science agrees it's the best all natural cure.

Keep in mind that any movement you do beats the couch, and while you're healing you will have limitations, but don't let them stop you. There is always something you can do and we'll show you how in this section.

- Are you ready to feel better fast?
- Need more motivation?

What if I told you that exercise could fortify your immune system to fight against future cancers, make you feel healthier after treatments and reduce pain and extreme fatigue? If that's not enough to get you moving, science agrees that exercise boosts the tumor-fighting ability of chemotherapy. Study after study has proven it to be true. Exercise is just plain good for you.

Exercise has even more benefits for cancer patients undergoing treatments. Exercise combined with chemotherapy can shrink tumors even more than chemotherapy alone.

While exercise has been prescribed and recommended for its physical and psychological benefits, we now know it's an integral part of treatment. Exercise is one of the most important aspects of treatment and needs to be prioritized as a part of integrated therapies.

Most of us will do whatever it takes to get rid of the cancer, but we forget that, in the long run, it's not cancer that affects us the worst. Rather, it's the side effects of the treatments that do the most harm. Smart exercise can help offset some of these negative side effects.

115

One of the most important aspects of exercise is muscle retention, which keeps us strong physically and mentally. However, the muscle that needs to be protected the most is our heart.

IMMUNE SYSTEM FORTIFYING AND HEART HEALTH HELPING

We can't forget that our heart is a muscle and if we don't exercise it daily, and nourish it with the right food, it atrophies. That's what makes us tired and weak. Exercise also helps offset the toxic effects of some medications. The most surprising evidence is the tumor shrinkage and pain reduction due to endorphins (happy hormones) that help offset the pain, making it easier to manage. If pain medication is needed, it makes it more efficient, as exercise helps it reach areas of the body that have poor circulation.

Who knew something as simple as moving could help nutrients or medication be metabolized?

The truth is, the more active you are, the stronger you'll be, and your chances of survival are greater. Did we mention physical activity is also helpful in lowering body weight and reducing the risk of heart disease and diabetes, just to name a few?

The best news is that anything you do that requires movement is going to bring you benefits. It doesn't matter if you've never exercised before in your life prior to today. A tailored home fitness plan will help you feel better faster than anything you'll ever do. What stops most people, is they don't know where to start, or what to do. Staying strong is easier than you think.

> **Exercise also helps to create a healthy appetite for patients who are struggling with eating, which allows them to *muscle waste*—making them feel weak and depressed.**

THREE STEPS THAT WILL KEEP YOU STRONG

Important Note: Proceed with happy caution, and be sure to speak to your cancer team and ask them about your limitations, as well as when the best time to start is. Since every case is different, and we all have different needs, only your doctor knows for sure what is best for you, and you must listen to your body.

More is not better when it comes to exercise. Think of exercise as your prescription for better health and healing. You wouldn't dream of taking more medication than prescribed, so exercise should be treated the same. In fact, if you get excessive and compulsive, you can hurt your immune system, and this plan is all about boosting it, and making you feel happier.

> **Get yourself a pedometer or Fit Bit to track your steps and time all day long. It will make you feel like something good is happening, and that's always a plus.**

Step #1: Get Up and Move Every Hour—Sitting still for extended periods of time increases your risk of heart failure. Since inactivity also contributes to obesity, sitting too long is not a good thing for your entire body.

Science agrees that a simple stroll can help reduce cancer risk. Exercise helps regulate the hormones, estrogen, and insulin; the two hormones that may lead to cancer growth. If you aren't feeling up to it, or you don't have time to fit a 30-minute walk into your day, it's just as beneficial to divide up your workout into shorter bursts.

On a low day, you may need to walk for 5 minutes every hour. Believe it or not that will provide you 10,000 steps, or 60 minutes (if you walked 5 minutes every hour, in a 12-hour day). It doesn't matter whether you stroll around your house, hospital or outside. Some people even walk in place. It all counts.

If you're well enough, you can bike, swim or perform any moderate activity. It is important to accept your new normal, and go slower and easier.

Here's a special note to gym warriors out there. The need to prove you are in control over cancer may cause you to climb outrageous mountains like join Cross Fit, or go on Mud Runs or Warrior Dashes until you can't move. This is not good for your immune system, so stick to your exercise prescription for best results, so you stay healthy.

Keep in mind that your doctor knows best when it comes to starting, or resuming, your exercise. Talk with your doctor regarding gauging where to start, and how long it should take to get back to the fitness level where you left off.

Even if you were working out right up until your surgery, it's important to start back slowly. The rule of thumb is if you were unable to exercise for 3 weeks, it should take you 3 weeks to get back to the level you left off. If you push too hard, too fast, you'll end up either hurting yourself or delaying the healing process. It doesn't matter how fit and strong you were.

Cancer and surgery put a lot of stress on your body, and you need to focus all of your efforts on healing.

I had surgery on my lower leg, and I didn't want to place too much pressure on it, which might have resulted in the wound breaking open or increasing the duration of swelling and pain. Immediately after my surgery, on the advice of my surgeon, I rested for a week. I then biked gently for 15 minutes every day.

Prior to my melanoma surgery I was biking or walking for 60 minutes daily. Once the stitches were removed and I was given the green signal by my surgeon, I gradually increased my regimen until I was back to my normal routine in about 4 weeks.

Since melanoma can strike any body part, and the exact type of surgery you have may vary, you must discuss the resumption of exercise with your doctor and come up with a safe plan. If you are okay to walk, start slowly by walking for 20 minutes, 3–4 days weekly, building up to daily exercise. You can walk outside or slowly on a treadmill. Mall walks work too if needed.

You lose a lot of muscle mass after major surgery. You need to get that muscle back. Not just for looks, but also for injury prevention. If your core is weak, you're more vulnerable to back issues, and could hurt yourself.

Staying physically active helps you stay emotionally stable. After surgery and treatments, you will want to put cancer behind you. I know I needed to promise and remind myself to never to give into self-pity. I had to focus on my kids and stay physically and spiritually fit to get through the rough times.

I woke up early to do 10 minutes of stretching, and 10 minutes of strengthening, every day. I also walked as much as I could every day by taking the stairs whenever I felt up to it and parked further away for shopping and appointments than necessary.

I also made it a point to stroll down every aisle when I shopped, just to add in extra steps to help offset the extra rest and sitting I needed while healing. I feel better emotionally when I feel better physically. Staying fit or focusing on fitness makes us feel empowered, and that we can handle anything that comes our way.

Once your body heals, you can increase your exercise to help you continue to gain strength. We might not be able to cure cancer with exercise, but it's the best way to fight back.

Finding your inner fitness beyond appearance and maintaining strength during treatments can be a struggle. Medications can drain away your energy and leave you nauseated. Trust that exercise is active meditation and will help you get the blood flowing after surgery. Physiologically it makes you feel stronger because you're helping your body heal.

Step #2: Boost Your Mood and Health in 10 Minutes—This simple routine builds strength while tightening and toning your body.

Notes: Be careful not to tire yourself out beforehand, and be patient with yourself. This isn't forever.

These moves are safe for most, 1 month after surgery (always check with your doctor first). Start slowly and rest when needed.

Perform 1–2 sets of each move. Aim for 10–12 repetitions, building up to performing each movement for 1 minute, rest if needed, and then move on. Repeat the circuit 2–3 times, 2–3 days per week. Short on time, or not feeling well enough to do all of the moves? Choosing one movement each day will allow you to feel stronger.

Warm up first by walking around your house, or in place, for 1–2 minutes until you begin to feel warm.

- **Chair Squats**
  Stand with feet shoulder-width apart, arms crossed over your chest to keep posture straight and squat down, sticking your butt out behind you until you're seated in a chair. Using your heels, push yourself back up. Protect your knees by keeping your knee back behind your toe, and don't allow your knee to go over or past your toes.

- **Upper Body Booster Wall or Counter Top Push-Ups**
  Stand facing your kitchen counter top or door jam. Lean forward and place your hands on the edge(s), keeping your back and arms straight. Bend elbows to lower your chest to the counter or door frame opening. Slowly push back up as you straighten your arms.

- **Bent Over Row Back Strengthener**
  Seated in a chair, bend over from your waist while keeping a flat back. Hold dumbbells in your hands and lower the dumbbells to the floor. Pull them back up, as if starting a lawn mower. This move can also be done standing up and leaning on a wall, supporting yourself with one arm, and working one side at a time to accommodate your limitations.

- **Core Strengthener Bicycle Crunches**
  Lie on your back with your hands behind your head for support. Be careful not to pull at your neck. Raise your shoulders off the floor and bend your knees in toward your chest as if riding a bike. Alternate bringing one knee up to touch the opposite elbow. Do this to each side, performing a bicycling motion.

- **Strong Core—Better Back Pelvic Tilts**
  Lay on your back with your knees bent. Flatten your back against the floor by tightening your abdominal muscles and bend/curl your pelvis up slightly. Hold for a 10-count, and repeat. Don't forget to exhale.

Step #3: Stretch Your Way to Faster Healing—Exercise is one of the best ways to meditate. Some people think of meditation as the yogi position of cross-legged, hands together, eyes closed and letting out the "Om" sound. However; many survivors, including myself, become so anxious, physically and mentally when trying to meditate this way.

Unless you're practiced at it, you become anxious, and focus is difficult. Your mind wanders and meditation becomes one more place of worry and anxious thoughts.

In my 25+ years in the nutrition and fitness industry, I have worked with countless people, some of whom were celebrities, and this was often the case. What I found was that the more they focused on the exercise movements, the more they performed the moves correctly, instead of trying not to obsess on their issues. Their minds began to meditate into the rhythm of the exercise.

It is very difficult to blank out your mind, especially when your health and well-being is the issue. Our thoughts are not meant to come to a screeching halt, but rather to learn to stay conscious and be able to escape uncomfortable situations and circumstances by focusing on something other than what's bothering us.

It's a good thing to meet your body and mind where it is and accept it, versus shutting yourself off from it.

Daily stretching is the secret to a healthier, less achy body. Aches and pains are your body's way of letting you know it's out of balance, and you need to stretch. Recovering from surgery or treatments is much harder on the body than we realize, and all the sitting still and inactivity can make our body ache.

While we rest, our body rusts. Movement helps grease our body, improving circulation all over. This delivers the nutrients your body needs to heal. Movement and stretching also help remove chemicals that may interfere with healing and will help you recover faster. You should make stretching your active daily meditation, so you become more in touch with your body and yourself.

Stretching is great for those days you're not feeling well while you're waiting for the doctor, or going for your treatment. So distract yourself and do it until you feel better. Besides, tight muscles are a sign of a stressed body. It will make you more prone to injury. Stretching your body and your mind is the best way to prevent this.

The three moves on the next page are movements everyone should do each day to keep the body and mind in working order.

- **The Back Fixer**
  Lying flat on your back and keeping one knee bent, raise the opposite leg straight to a 90-degree angle. Hold for 8–10 seconds. Repeat on the other side. Perform 2–3 times, or as needed until you feel a release.

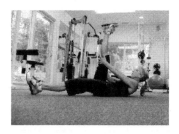

- **The Butt Stretch and Hip Opener**
  Lay on your back, bend one leg at 90-degree angle, place the ankle of opposite leg/foot in front of your knee. Pull back to feel a gentle stretch in your butt and hips. Hold while gently pulling back for 8–10 seconds. Repeat on the other side. Perform this 2–3 times, or as needed until you feel a release.

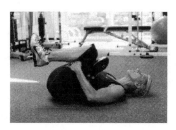

- **The Total Release Stretch**
  Raise your arms above your head and gently lean to each side (you can also do this lying flat on the floor), extending in each direction. Hold each position for 8–10 seconds. Tilt to the right and hold for 8–10 seconds and repeat on the left. Repeat 2–3 times, or as needed until you feel a release.

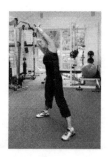

This move rocks because you can do it in bed or while in the shower (be careful), or anytime you feel anxious. I do this stretch standing while waiting for the doctor instead of focusing on the fear factor.

Keep in mind that wherever your thoughts go, your body will follow. Stretching helps to relax your mind and your body, but you will need to surrender to the stretch by focusing on your breathing, and making sure you are exhaling. You'll notice that your breath drives the move. Exhaling makes your body release and let go.

Need a quick fix? Feeling extra anxious? Exhale hard by lifting your shoulders and forcing your breath out hard.

BAD DAY QUICK FIX: Play your favorite relaxing song while you stretch. No matter what's going on you'll feel better; resulting in your total body, mind, and spirit stretching.

"We pay a heavy price for our fear of failure. It is a powerful obstacle to growth. It assures the progressive narrowing of the personality and prevents exploration and experimentation. There is no learning without some difficulty and fumbling. If you want to keep on learning, you must keep on risking failure — all your life. "
- John W. Gardner

ELEVEN

Positive Outlook | Spiritual Belief

Learning How to Live a Wholesome Lifestyle with, or After Cancer
While you are being treated for cancer, it's not just your body being attacked by drugs, radiation, or surgery. Your mind is also being attacked by fear and doubt, shaking your faith like never before.

The only way to fight fear and win is with faith, through power prayer.

> **When fear comes knocking at your door answer it with faith. What other choice do you have? It's one or the other. Which one will you choose? You always have a choice no matter how dark things seem. You can't allow dread or fear into your life. Fear and worry produces more fear and worry. Prayer and peace produces more prayer and peace. You need to choose joy and peace now more than ever.**
>
> **This is the true essence of using the power of your body, mind and spirit. It will set you free no matter what happens to your body.**

As discussed earlier, there are ways to get your body prepared for surgery so that you'll recover more quickly, but what about your mental and spiritual health? To heal, you need your body, mind and spirit in perfect alignment. They all need to be in agreement with each other.

Thinking about it this way helped me to understand why I couldn't treat my body carelessly, and continue to think negatively. It just doesn't work. We are only human, and this alignment isn't easy when you're scared out of your mind.

There are lots of hocus pocus self-help techniques, but, to be honest, I've never liked any of them. I've tried them, but I never left a session feeling safe, whole and fulfilled. The truth is, I was afraid to sit still and feel my feelings. I've learned that facing my fears is mandatory when it comes to actual healing.

With most of the self-help techniques, the intent is to escape from our horrible reality and enter into a place of nothingness bliss. This is great, except for one problem—we always return to the real world where our problems are waiting for us.

The only way for us to heal on the inside is to give ourselves permission to feel our way through, and to allow ourselves the time and space to process those uncomfortable feelings. When we do that, our feelings no longer have control over us. The bottom line is—you've got to feel it to heal it.

I challenge you to face your fears and fight back with faith. Allow your real feelings to surface, let them show. Be fearless when showing your affections (not just the ugly sentiments), and you'll live a deeper, happier more fulfilling life.

The battle is won in your mind, and it all starts with feeling our emotions. These techniques will:

- Decrease stress levels
- Boost immune function
- Decrease pain
- Help in faster recovery after procedures
- Aid in fewer side effects from chemotherapy
- Lessen anxiety, which decreases symptoms
- Improve mood and lessen suppression of emotions, which leads to increased feeling of wellness or well-being.

When we worry about nothing because we pray about everything, we can finally relax, which helps us gain perspective. We feel less overwhelmed by cancer and treatment. Praying during difficult times automatically relaxes you (you're still conscious and present, and you're expressing your feelings). This begins the emotional healing process. When we pray, the stressor loses its control over us.

I'm going to show you a few power prayer techniques that I've learned as a chaplain that can help you cope. These techniques improve recovery after treatments, as well as in any difficult circumstance.

Praying when we are stressed helps to lower cortisol and other metabolic mediators that may fuel cancer growth.

RELAX YOUR MIND AND YOU'LL RELAX YOUR BODY

Find a Quiet Place: Our environment plays a significant role in helping us relax. It's harder to relax in a noisy office or a part of your home filled with people. You need a quiet place without interruption where you feel safe and secure.

Most of us have a favorite chair, or it may be your bed. Relaxing in bed with my dogs and kids is my favorite place to be on earth. When all else fails, you can use Muscle Relaxation Techniques and Guided Imagery to imagine you are in that location. These are a great help during treatments when all you can do is think.

Almost every survivor I speak to say they visualized a blue ocean and focused on the sound of the waves. Whatever works for you, go visit that place. I like to bring earphones if the sounds around me are making me tense. I listen to the songs that take me to another place and relax.

Relax Your Breathing: Breathing deeply and slowly maximizes the flow of oxygen into the blood, promoting a relaxed feeling. Practice inhaling deeply and exhale as slowly as you can.

You can slow your breathing down by inhaling deeply and exhaling as slowly as possible, relaxing your body. Tell your body to wilt as you slowly exhale, especially the tight muscles, so you're totally relaxed. Take your time and make as many relaxing breaths as you need, until you feel totally relaxed.

A cleansing breath is when you exhale hard while visualizing any ache or pain you may have has left your body, as well as any negative thoughts. Each time you exhale visualize all of your stress leaving. If your mind races, say the Serenity Prayer: "God grant me the serenity to accept the things I cannot change, the courage to change the things I can, and the wisdom to know the difference."

Relax Each and Every Muscle: Relaxing your muscles is as easy as thinking about each muscle group and relaxing the tension as you move from one area to another.

Begin with your feet, think about your toes and ask them to relax. As you exhale and release the stress, progress to your ankle, then your calf, knee, and so on until you have reached your head.

If you find that you are holding tension in one particular area, stay there, breathe deeply, and ask the pain what it represents.

Don't be surprised if you begin crying or feeling very emotional, as most times these pains are a sign that we are holding stress in our bodies, and we only need to relax.

We can train our brain not to feel pain by breathing in slowly and deeply, and exhaling out all of the toxic thoughts and feelings.

Still feel uptight? Go get a massage. Touch, whether through a hug, massage or otherwise, is an excellent way to release anti-stress hormones that make our body feel good all over.

NEED A SPIRITUAL DETOXIFICATION?
Try this 10-second spiritual detox:

- Ask yourself if there is something specific causing you to worry
- Give yourself 10 seconds to think about it, and then STOP
- What thoughts came up? This may not relax you right away, but it begins the process of accepting what we can't change, and it helps you figure out what feelings you need to process.
- The next step is to talk to your friends or cancer support group so they can help you handle these feelings. The minute you open up and talk, you will feel relief.

TRAIN YOUR BRAIN NOT TO FEEL PAIN WITH GUIDED IMAGERY
Have you ever heard the saying: "Where your head goes, your body follows"? It's true. Guide the images in your mind, and you guide your thoughts.

Guided imagery is the use of mental images to help influence how your body feels. You're just training your imagination to take you to a less stressful place.

Remember the days when you used to daydream when you were in school? Guided imagery is exactly that. Our thoughts, and the images that flow from our imagination influence our emotion and spirit, as well as our body.

Remember the last time you were excited to go on vacation, and you couldn't stop thinking about it and all you were going to do there? You just proved to yourself that you can do it. Now apply that to your cancer treatment. Picture yourself feeling relaxed and your entire body responding to treatment.

You can learn to use this same kind of mind power to produce calming and healing responses in your body. Instead of thinking about your cancer and treatments, which escalate your fears and anxiety, start retraining your brain to think of better thoughts. Practice every day, so you're a pro when you need these skills to help you the most.

Visualize flipping the "on" switch every time you need to think positive, soothing, happy thoughts. When the negative thoughts enter your mind, flip the switch "on".

Guided imagery is just controlled daydreaming. Practice these techniques daily, or at least 3 times weekly, so your skills are sharp when you need them most.

When all else fails, fake it until you make it or go play with your dog or kids. You'll quickly forget what was worrying you. Never underestimate the power of distraction.

Guided imagery can be used to reduce anxiety, decrease muscle tension and pain, ease sleep problems, speed healing and recovery, and most importantly give you a feeling of control over your body.

The physiological benefits of guided imagery have been documented in many studies. The most common and efficient techniques use positive mental images. Images such as powerful white light permeating every cell in your body, healing them and creating a feeling of bliss. Or visualize a cancer vacuum that sucks up and kills cancer cells.

Creating your creative visual is an excellent exercise to do daily to distract and retrain your brain to think right thoughts, vs. fear and worry. It's a process known to physiologists as restructuring, where you learn to replace anticipated negative thoughts with an image of the opposite effect.

Try to replace the fearful picture or thought with a pleasant feeling. Visualize that God has you in his arms, keeping you safe, or chemo is your friend and she (meaning chemo) is traveling through your body fixing things.

Keep playing these mind images and awareness until nausea passes. This might not sound natural, but it is just as easy to think happy thoughts as it is to think scary thoughts. You'll feel better when not focusing on the yucky stuff. Anyone can do this. All you have to do is decide to, and practice.

Wouldn't you like to feel less stress, free of anxiety, and more relaxed? This imagery exercise will strengthen your capacity to draw on your emotional resources. So get ready for some good memories to come up to the surface and surprise you with feelings of safety and calmness. Feelings like you're floating on air watching the movie of life, where you see every puppy, kitten or baby you've been touched by.

Maybe your mind will take you to that particular place where you feel like life is good. It's all governed by our mind's ability to leave, and by paying attention to our breath.

Breathing is one of the most powerful conscious influences you have over your nervous system. Remember to exhale hard, as it will release the stress. Go deep and take the time to appreciate these scenes with all of your senses.

- What does it smell like?
- What sounds can you hear?
- Can you feel the warm, safe sun on your sun-blocked face?
- What are you wearing?
- Can you touch and feel anything?
- What time of day is it?
- Are you alone, or with people you love? Maybe your dog is by your side?

Now take notice of how your body feels. Enjoy this feeling and stay there as long as you need to. Have fun with this if you need to. Make it work for you so you can use these skills to get to bliss quickly and whenever you want.

Whenever you need to travel to your safe place, start with your breath. Allow your breaths to deepen and feel your body getting heavy. Your shoulders are dropping, and any tightening you feel is now being released. Close your eyes and allow your body to go totally limp, including your mind.

How well do you feel now?

Imagery worked better than pain medication for Marcia, who fought and won stage 3 melanoma. She had to endure multiple surgeries, and her anxiety took its toll on her health. In fact, the side effects from her overly anxious mind were worse and more debilitating than the recovery from the surgery.

Marcia knew there had to be a better way to deal with all of this so she began to practice these guided imagery mind meditations daily until she mastered her mind and started to laugh again.

Not only did Marcia start laughing, which is good for our bodies because it releases happy hormones, she was also able to eat regular, nutritious foods. This gave her the energy she needed to live her life and enjoy it.

REDUCING THE STRESS EFFECT OF SURGERY

Are you feeling scared before surgery or treatment? Most of us are afraid because the unknown can be scary when we are worried about the change in our bodies. Death, pain, getting a poor diagnosis, or not being able to live normally or being disabled also contribute.

Powerlessness, my least favorite emotion, is the worst fear. Everyone I speak to shares this feeling. Remember the stress effect? Stress undermines our bodies, which directly affects how we heal.

Your doctor will prepare you for the physical aspects of surgery—explaining what will happen. They may not realize how scary that sounds, so you need to prepare yourself by developing your mind. You do this by prayer, and the relaxation exercises mentioned earlier. This gets your body, mind, and soul aligned with each other for faster/quantum healing. If your recovery is slow, practice the steps listed below again, until you're on the road to healing.

FIVE STEPS TO QUICKLY REDUCE STRESS – STRENGTHEN YOUR FAITH MUSCLES AND CLING TO PEACE

These simple solutions have helped countless survivors reduce post-operative stress, reduce post-operative pain, and calm nervous jitters. Feeling peaceful is important because it strengthens your immune system and creates a miraculous bio-chemistry that enhances healing.

1. Organize your miracle prayer network, or social support group. Avoid toxic people.
2. Relax to feel peaceful—Peace out
3. Visualize your healing
4. Worry about nothing, pray about everything
5. Use your words. Speak healing words only

Need help? Don't have a network? Join a group, or you can buy guided imagery or a healing statement CD, to do the work for you.

This worked so well for Mary J. Mary met with her anesthesiologist prior to surgery, and asked him to repeat her healing statements as she was being sedated. Doing this reinforced the relaxation effect, and because her anxiety was reduced, she needed less post-operative pain medication. All these made her feel healthy and well, more quickly.

Remember, you can begin visualizing your recovery right now by performing these exercises. Do what Mary J has done for yourself as well. If you're too shy to ask, surround yourself with family and friends who love you, and can calm you before surgery.

I suggest using a guided imagery CD or practicing your mind meditations every day for 2 weeks before surgery. Perform them on your way to the operating room to reduce anticipation anxiety. Perform them when you're receiving chemo to help alleviate nausea.

Make this positive power your new healthy. Continue to practice these techniques every day, especially after treatment. Imagery/mind games are the best way to reduce stress from surgery.

> **KEEPING THE MIND AND BODY IN HARMONY MAKES TREATMENT MORE EFFECTIVE.**

TAKING CARE OF THE CAREGIVER

Not everyone who reads this book is a melanoma patient. The reader might be someone taking care of a patient with melanoma. This is for them.

Have you ever listened to a flight attendant when she is giving emergency instructions? The first thing she teaches parents or caregivers is to put their oxygen mask on first before helping their children or others in need. There is a good reason. If they are not okay, they can't take care of anyone else. The same goes for those in a caregiving position. Taking care of your health is just as important as the patient's needs.

Caregivers are angels on earth. All of the caregivers I've interviewed were the most patient people I have ever met. If you are a caregiver and you are reading this: GOD BLESS YOU. If not, good for you for showing concern for the caregivers needs.

You cannot give what you do not possess. So take the time to fill your cup so that you can pour out. The housework can wait. The mess or the dust will be there when you can return to it. Take time for yourself, and you'll be better able to care for your patient or loved one.

Recovery time offers both patients and caregivers a unique opportunity to invest more in relationship and love.

I took care of my grandfather while he was recovering from heart surgery, and it was one of the hardest things I have ever done. It was also one of the most rewarding experiences in my life. First, I had to learn how to take care of myself, which wasn't easy.

It's not the big expensive vacations that offer the most bonding opportunities. Rather, it's the moments we catch making a meal together or enjoying a cup of tea while reminiscing about the good old days.

Take the time to sit and enjoy each other's company, and don't worry so much about how perfect the food is, or the day's details. The dust will be there after you're done enjoying each other. Relationships always come first.

I learned many life lessons from hospice nurses while spending time with my dad there. I felt so strongly about these particular pivotal moments that I went on to become a Chaplain. Here are tips from caregivers around the United States.

- **Pray about Everything**, and worry about nothing. Everything will be just fine.
- **Put Your "Oxygen Mask" On First**. Take care of yourself. Be sure to get plenty of rest, eat healthily, and don't forget to exercise your body, and relax your mind.
- **Be Patient.**
  Rose C – *"Love is patient. A triple dose of patience and prayer!"*
- **Let Your Love Flow.** Show your love, and give kisses and hugs.
  Dan M – *"Don't forget to hug them and tell them you love them. It's easy to forget to do the most important thing. Express how much we love them. Try not to get caught up in all of the things you have to do."*
- **Stay Positive and Stay Strong.**
  Elizabeth – *"Stay positive and stay strong. You can do this. Nothing is impossible when you put your trust in God. I know this one can be hard, but a positive outlook makes the day-to-day a little easier."*
- **Listen.**
  Vinny M – *"Be a good listener. Listen to their stories. They are amazing. And, listen closely to hear what they might be trying to tell you but are too afraid."*
- **Trust Your Instincts.**
  Lisa – *"If something doesn't feel right, it probably isn't. These gentle nudges (aka: "gut" feelings) are God's way of letting us know something is wrong. Trust your inner voice and ask questions until you feel relieved."*
- **Laugh Out Loud Every Day.**
  Janet D – *"Try to keep your sense of humor. Laughter is good for the soul and is the best stress reliever on the planet."*
- **Get Support For You.**
  Eileen L – *"Join a support group. The knowledge that you are not the only one going through this is valuable, and people learn from each other."*
  Tracy L – *"You aren't doing either of you any favors by struggling alone. There is strength in numbers."*

- **Get Organized.**
  Gail F – *"Make a medical binder in the event of an emergency. Include family phone numbers, names, addresses, Social Security numbers, all medications and time of day they're taken. Include any allergies, or note that there are none. List any previous medical issues, such as stroke, etc., and date of such. Include the health insurance and Medicare or Medicaid cards, and other identifying information. I had to take my mom to the hospital a few times. I had the binder with me because in an emergency situation you forget things. Let go and let God. He has you covered!"*

THE HEALING POWER OF SLEEP

SLEEP IS THE MOST UNDERESTIMATED WEAPON IN YOUR FIGHT

When was the last time you went to bed early and slept so well that you woke up feeling rejuvenated and optimistic? Maybe you felt peaceful and grounded, and you even laughed more throughout the day? You might have even noticed that your skin had a youthful glow, and your body ached less?

That incredible feeling was the miraculous healing power of a good night's sleep. When we sleep soundly, our body's healing night shift turns on. Its job is to release miracle healing chemicals and hormones. I'll get back to these miracle workers in a minute. First, it's important to understand why these might not be released.

Sometimes when we need sleep the most, it's the hardest to get. Ask any survivor and they will all agree it's almost impossible to get a good night's sleep in the hospital, or during treatments.

Doctors make their rounds at 5 a.m. or 6 a.m., waking people and disrupting sleep patterns. Interruptions are expected whether to check vital signs or check on patients who may be unstable. Not to mention the non-sleepers who like to watch television into the wee hours of the morning, and usually have it so loud they can hear it in the next state. These types of interruptions get on our nerves—literally.

Cancer brings a lot of stress with it, and our nervous systems are already under attack. The added weight of the treatments and hospital stays adds to this. Our nervous system is taxed to the limit, and one of the best ways to calm and soothe it is sleep.

Sleep is the miraculous healing time where our bodies heal, detoxify. The best part is our minds shut down (hopefully) and reboot. Sometimes when we are stressed, it becomes harder to sleep because our mind is so over-taxed, which can cause racing thoughts that we sometimes can't turn off even when we are exhausted. That's the time we need it most.

The survivors I've interviewed said they would finally get to sleep, and a nurse would wake them up to see if they need sleep medication. Don't be afraid to ask that your room be in a quieter section of the hospital and that interruptions be limited (and don't forget to use the relaxation exercises discussed earlier).

You'll also want to limit light exposure. This includes the lights from cell phones, televisions, laptops and all types of lighting. They interrupt sleep hormone production. All these impair your body from making enough melatonin, which is the hormone that helps you sleep.

I'm sure you know all too well, or firsthand, that cancer and its treatments cause an extreme level of fatigue, and that your sleep needs are dramatically increased. Sleeping is miraculous because it will improve these issues more than you realize. You should note that if your sleep has been interrupted for a while, it may take you a while to feel substantially better, but I can assure you that you will.

Prioritize getting more sleep, and take some time to pay into your sleep budget. You'll see drastic changes in your body, mind, and spirit.

It's important to note that while you're undergoing treatments like chemotherapy that cause pain, you may not have any control over waking up frequently during the night. That's nothing a few 20-minute naps won't fix. Be sure to nap early in the day, so you don't interrupt sleep at night.

For general health, we need at least 7–8 hours of sleep for our bodies to heal on a good day. When we are undergoing cancer treatments, or trying to keep our immune systems working at maximum efficiency, sleep becomes even more important. Our need increases, bringing our sleep numbers to 9–12 hours per day.

It's important to know this about yourself if you're like me and have a built-in alarm clock that goes off at 4:30 a.m. every day. Create a sleep budget, and stick to it. The new normal for you should be to make your bedtime be about the number of hours you need, vs. the time on the clock.

Listen to your body, and it will most likely tell you that it's sleep time as soon as the sun goes down. That's your body's natural biorhythm designed to keep you healthy. Now the stakes are even higher, so go to bed earlier so you can get the required sleep. The whole day is brighter when you've had enough rest.

Now you know why hospitals serve dinner so early. They expect you to go to sleep early. They also know that you shouldn't eat 3 hours before bedtime, as it will disrupt your sleep and your body's healing processes. That's the last thing you need when fighting cancer.

Don't be afraid to let well-wishing visitors know that you need them to come earlier, to allow you to doze off early. And that program on TV can be watched anytime with technology today. You'll enjoy it even more when rested.

Boosting Immunity and Our Biological Sleep Clock

You may be thinking, biological sleep clock? What's that? It's just another way of describing or naming your body's natural circadian rhythms.

Circadian rhythms are physical, mental and behavioral changes that follow a roughly 24-hour cycle, responding primarily to light and darkness in your environment.

Disrupting nature's circadian rhythm interferes with your sleep, and you can be the culprit in this, as it stops the natural healing process. When darkness falls, your pineal gland, located in the brain, increases its melatonin production. It releases in response to the decreased levels of light under normal circumstances when we are young and healthy. However, life and busy schedules take their toll on this process.

Typically when the sun sets, it signals melatonin to begin flowing. As your melatonin levels begin to rise, you start to feel sleepy. As you fall asleep, it flows faster. This faster pace of melatonin causes a surge, and melatonin becomes even more powerful.

If your sleep is interrupted, or you decide to stay up late instead, you disrupt this incredible healing process. The damage can last for a long time.

This miraculous melatonin pump is critical because its potential is so high that it becomes a powerful cancer fighter. It may even protect you from whatever comes your way; from the common cold or virus to the everyday aches and pains.

This circadian rhythm is a part of every cell in your body. In cancer cells, the rhythm is out of sync with healthy cells.

The outcome of chemotherapy may have a lot to do with these abnormal circadian rhythms. There have been studies that have shown that using drugs in the morning, or evening, can make a difference in the effectiveness, as well as how severe the side effects are.

Side effects from drugs may seem less severe when they are given at the right time. Bottom line, the more rest and quality sleep you get, the better you'll cope physically, mentally and spiritually. Remember you're fighting to win.

Back to the miracle worker called melatonin—the natural secret to a good night's sleep. Researchers discovered some of melatonin's miraculous healing properties, and this is why melatonin gets such red-carpet treatment from the media. Television personalities, news anchors, as well as doctors, suffer the most with sleep issues due to their sleep schedules disrupted by their job hours.

Here is why melatonin is so popular. Melatonin has been used in Europe for decades because it helps us recover from jet lag. It's a safe, natural alternative to sleeping pills. While melatonin's job is to promote drowsiness, so you fall asleep faster, it also has superhero properties you need to know.

For starters, better quality sleep means a turbocharged immune system. A turbocharged immune system means protection from cancer.

Melatonin is a potent antioxidant. Antioxidants are those powerful defenders that protect us from free radicals by making them incapable of damaging your cells and DNA. This type of harm has been shown to increase your risk of cancer. Less melatonin means our DNA is more prone to cancer-causing mutations.

Melatonin has been shown in some models to inhibit tumor growth. I suggest that anyone who has trouble sleeping, or works odd hours that might interrupt circadian rhythms, take 3–5 milligrams of melatonin.

Melatonin's superhero properties don't stop there. Melatonin has been known to:

- May stop new blood vessels from growing into tumors, which slows down the rate at which they grow and divide, preventing tumors from invading and spreading.
- Melatonin may also enhance the tumor-fighting power of vitamin D and increases its ability to stop tumor growth. Melatonin makes vitamin D's tumor-fighting abilities 20–100 times stronger.
- Supplementing with melatonin may enhance chemotherapy's effectiveness by increasing its capacity to kill tumors, decreasing the size of the tumors.
- Melatonin may provide protection from the harmful side effects of chemotherapy. Chemotherapy is commonly toxic to several components in the blood. Platelets, which help in blood clotting, are particularly vulnerable. Chemotherapy usually reduces the number of

platelets in the blood, which increases the risk of bleeding problems. On the other hand, melatonin protects the platelets and helps keep their numbers up. The researchers found that when melatonin was given to patients receiving chemotherapy, the number of platelets in their blood remained normal. These patients had fewer toxic side effects from the drugs, which included fewer mouth ulcers, and less damage to their nervous systems and hearts.

- Research also shows that if you go to bed early, before 10 p.m., your melatonin rises to the highest possible and most powerful levels during sleep. However, if you go to bed late, you're working against nature and interfering with its healing process. Keep in mind, melatonin likes darkness, so if you sleep with a TV or computer on, you prevent melatonin from rising to its full potential.

The Secret Powers of a Good Night's Sleep

Sleep is your secret weapon to win the fight. Melatonin is only one part of the immune boosting/cancer protection you gain during sleep.

Your sleep patterns govern changes in your immune system that either help to boost immunity to fight off disease or lower it, allowing the disease to take over.

You need sleep to charge your immune system sufficiently so it can fight tumors with a substance called tumor necrosis factor. This is a natural biological weapon that destroys tumors. It's a powerful immune booster that can only be produced during sleep. Your immune system creates 10-times more tumor necrosis factor when you're asleep than when you're awake.

When you sleep, your immune system also releases NK cells, or natural killer cells. You can think of these cells as superhero cells that kill tumor cells and any other undesirable cells that invade your body. If you don't get enough sleep, your immune system won't respond to commands to make more of these potent NK cells. Researchers agree that without adequate sleep, the number of NK cells goes down significantly.

Sleep Facts:

- The best sleep cycle is 10 p.m.–6 a.m.
- Sleep less and you also increase your risk of diabetes, high blood pressure, and weight gain, while disease creeps in
- Lack of sleep has been known to cause:
  - pain
  - depression
  - symptoms

o   possibly initiate cancers

What happens when you can't sleep? When you can't sleep, you feel stressed, even on a good day. This lack of sleep increases the production of cortisol, the stress hormone when melatonin should be working.

This creates the perfect storm for sleeping problems, which then take on a life of their own. This begins the chronic sleep problems a lot of us face, especially when we are under stress. A lot of people use sleeping pills, which only places a bandage on the problem.

Hopefully, you are now motivated to make sleep a priority in your life. Good quality sleep is imperative for balancing your hormonal systems and is crucial in making cancer treatment more effective.

The use of sleeping pills is also known to influence pain and increased depressive symptoms. However, people who sleep 6–8 hours had lower cortisol level.

TIPS FOR HEALTHY SLEEP

➢ **Don't exercise in the evening or too close to bedtime. Exercise is a stimulant.**
➢ **Don't drink alcohol; eat spicy or heavy foods that are hard to digest.**
➢ **Try to have your last meal of the day at least 3 hours before you sleep.**
➢ **Avoid all sources of caffeine late in the evening (Note: chocolate has caffeine).**
➢ **DO NOT go to bed with your laptop or iPad. The light from these affects your melatonin levels.**

STRESS AND MELANOMA

Studies have shown that there is a distinct correlation between a stressful event and the onset of melanoma. These events are significant life events like a death in the family of a partner, spouse or child; divorce, loss of a job or a serious accident.

While we are powerless to predict the onset, or indeed the course of these events, what we can and must do is to seek help (ideally professional) in dealing with these uniquely stressful events.

Friends, family, social or religious networks also play a crucial ancillary role in minimizing the ill effects of these events and help in maintaining the body's ability to fight off cancer.

How to Stay Physically, Mentally and Spiritually Strong to Boost Immunity

If you have been diagnosed with melanoma, or any cancer for that matter, you know firsthand how hard it is to stay positive and remain hopeful when your body is paralyzed with fear.

It's okay to feel every emotion from anger, denial, hopelessness and vulnerability. It's actually necessary to experience these feelings to process or work through them and begin the healing process.

If you take one thing away from this book, it should be to not keep these feelings to yourself. Talk to your doctor, who can help you put your fears into perspective. When we address fear head on, it loses its power over us and allows us to move forward into a place of physical, mental, and emotional healing.

The same way you have a cancer care team, you need a spiritual and emotional support system as well. It's imperative to grasp the truth fully that to heal, we need to address the disease from every aspect of our being. Physically, mentally and most importantly, the spiritual level.

Most of us treat healing and recovery in an upside down way. We will address every physical issue, show up for every doctor appointment, but what have you done for your spirit lately?

You see fear is the opposite of faith. Fear traumatizes, torments and makes us feel miserable and depressed. It makes you feel hopeless and helpless. These feelings will trap you on the pity pot, which is the loneliest place to be.

This is fear's game strategy and ultimately helps it win if you allow it in. Remember fear has no mercy. Fear wants you dwelling on the bad things.

The fight is won by choosing faith, and acting on it. You will miss out on joy, peace and physical, mental, and spiritual harmony if you choose fear vs. faith. Faith is a muscle, and you need to keep it strong by surrounding yourself with faithful, positive people.

Thinking positively, listening to uplifting music, and watching motivating movies like "Rocky", because you are who and with what you surround yourself. It's imperative that you spend time developing your faith muscles. You need to stay strong now more than ever.

This situation is temporary. Think of it as a faith upgrade, or an opportunity to overcome all your fears. It will bring you a victorious outcome in spirit, mind and body. You can live in freedom.

Even in the darkest of hours, you can always choose to look up. Here are the eight steps to happiness:

1. There is always something to be grateful for—find it. You're here now, right?
   One 14-year-old patient said, "I'm grateful for this bed. It is so comfortable."
2. Everything that happens is an opportunity for growth. Embrace it, and you'll experience why you are here on this earth.
3. Denial is a deal breaker. You've got to feel it to heal it. Don't deny that you're sick. Accept it so that you can move on. If you are religious, the power of prayer works. Create your support system/miracle prayer network and ask them to pray for you every day. I've met survivors who were atheists before they got sick, and each one said they could feel the prayers. Sometimes you don't know that God is all you need until God is all you have. If you are not surrounded by supportive people, seek council with clergy or a chaplain. You can submit online prayers. Your prayers still get heard, and you get the much-needed faith-lift.
4. Always choose faith over fear
5. Be boastful with yourself vs. blaming yourself. You can't go back and undo the things you've done in the past. Live in today and every time you want to blame yourself, boost yourself instead. Say positive things to yourself like, "I'm making the right decisions for me", or "I'm handling this well."
6. Live like you have run out of time
7. Say I love you to everyone
8. Hug more

Turn your mess into your mission. It's important to have a reason to get out of bed every day, especially when you're sick.

While we might be sick, we can protect our loved ones and help them avoid melanoma by practicing sun-safe habits and staying out of tanning beds.

Let your mission become your life's masterpiece.

What have you got to lose? You'll feel better and be happier.

DAILY POWER RELAXATION PRAYER:

I am physically healthy, mentally strong.

I can do all things.

I can now allow myself to relax.

Everything is okay.

It is easy for me to calm down.

I am safe.

All that's important is that I am relaxed.

Everything happens for my highest good.

I can afford to relax.

I can allow myself to enjoy this moment.

My will to relax is greater than any other thought.

I let go of stress with each breath I take.

This moment is perfect to relax.

Being relaxed is natural to me.

Letting go of stress is the best thing I can do right now.

I am able to relax whenever I choose to do so.

Book Closing

It is our hope that you will take care of yourself physically, mentally and spiritually and that you will be genuinely motivated to make your health the top priority in your life.

Be motivated and as active as possible in all these ways. Most importantly, have faith because without faith, we have nothing.

A PERSONAL MESSAGE FROM LISA LYNN

I don't know about you, but I am passionate and dedicated and can't sit back and watch people suffer. I've decided to donate every year to this particular research: Yale Melanoma Research Fund. It can save your life or the life of a loved one.

Scientists are continually learning new ways to put the brakes on cancer and hopefully stomp out melanoma, along with other cancers. Their challenge is to increase survival rates and ease this pointless suffering once and for all.

We can't do this alone, but with your help we can fight the battle and win. No donation is too small, and if each one of you contributes what you can, it can help make dreams become a reality.

Hope is achieved in the lab. Yale-New Haven Hospital's research is unique because of the dedicated Melanoma Specialists who are running it and devoting their lives to this mission.

Your donation, 100 percent, goes directly to research—not someone's pocket.

God bless you. Keep your faith muscles strong!

INDEX

S

sentinel node biopsy, 47, 48, 54, 58, 60, 61, 63, 64, 65, 75
shave biopsy, 41
SPF, 31, 32, 33, 34
Spitz nevus, 12
SUN BLOCK, 31
superficial spreading, 8

T

T cell, 85, 88, 89
TCR (T cell Receptor Therapy), 89
Trametinib, 82, 84

U

UPF, 33
UV index, 34
UVA, 29, 31, 33
UVB, 29, 31, 33
UVC, 29

V

Vemurafanib, 77, 82, 83, 84, 87

Y

Yervoy, 77, 85, 86